Addiction Recovery DIY:

Coloring Book with Motivational Quotes

For Stress Relief During Early Recovery

support@5Dmedia.org

Ordering Information: Quantity sales. Special discounts are available on quantity purchases by corporations, associations, and others. For details, contact the publisher at the address above.

Orders by U.S. trade bookstores and wholesalers. Please contact Big Distribution: orders@5dmedia.org or visit www.5DMedia.org.

Printed in the United States of America

Addiction Recovery DIY: Coloring Book with Motivational Quotes For Stress Relief During Early Recovery / K.J. Gordon

ISBN-10: 0-9989217-6-9
ISBN-13: 978-0-9989217-6-1

First Edition

This motivational coloring book was for created to support anyone in Detox or Addiction Recovery for relief at home, in a clinic or hospital, or during an extended stay at a residential rehab facility.

Getting and staying clean can be a stressful and lonely experience, with various challenges. Coloring is a relaxing technique that focuses the mind, similar to yoga and meditation. The repetition and simplicity can reduce your stress levels by slowing down your heart rate and breathing, and relaxing your muscles.

This combination of quieting the mind and coloring has been found helpful for those dealing with anxiety and other recovery related issues.

For additional encouragement, simply remove your favorite pages to display around the house with ease, as each coloring page is single sided and features a motivational quote.

If you think you may need additional help, or just someone to talk to, follow up on Instagram @AddictionRecoveryDIY or Facebook.com/DrugRecovery.

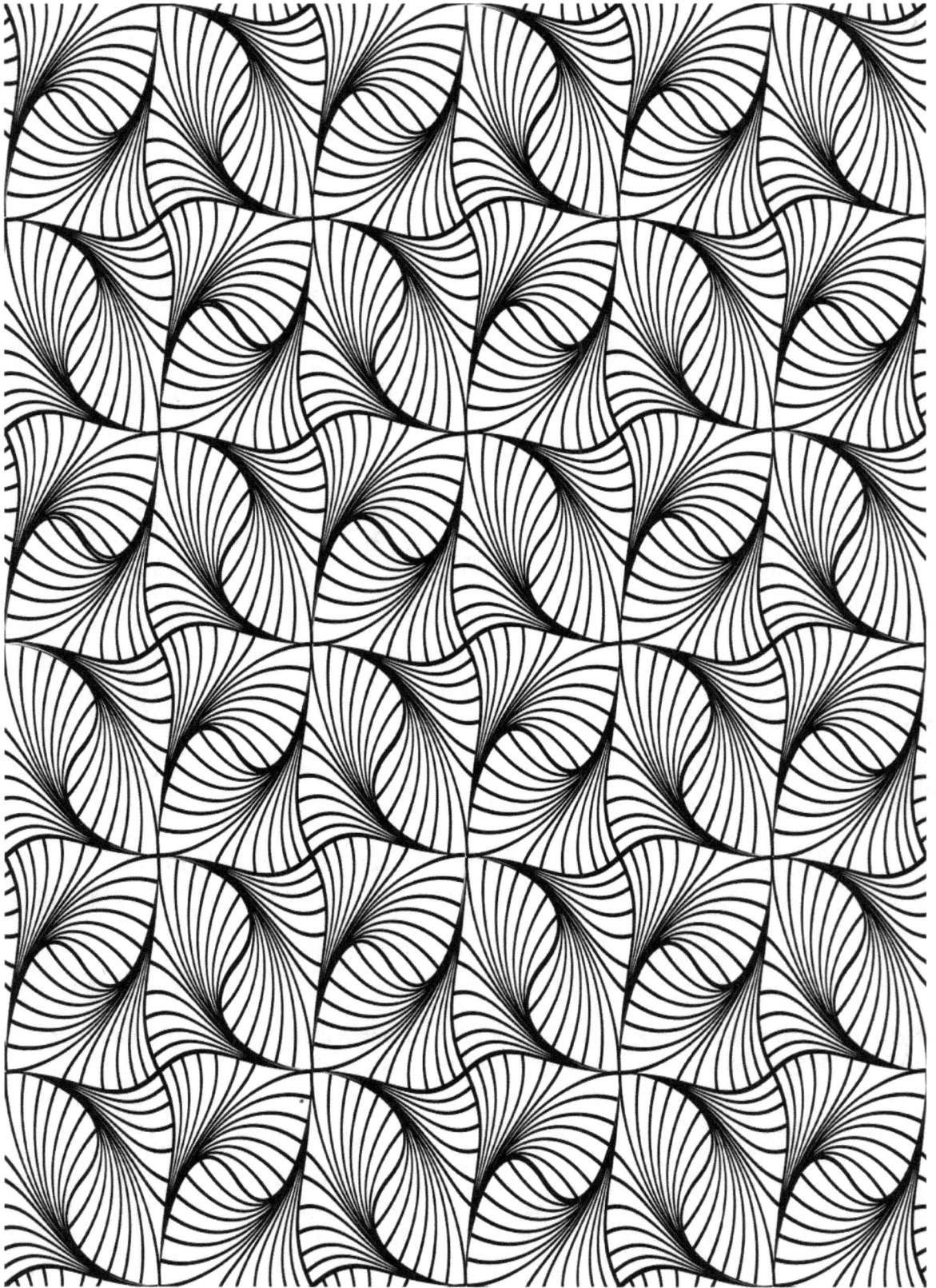

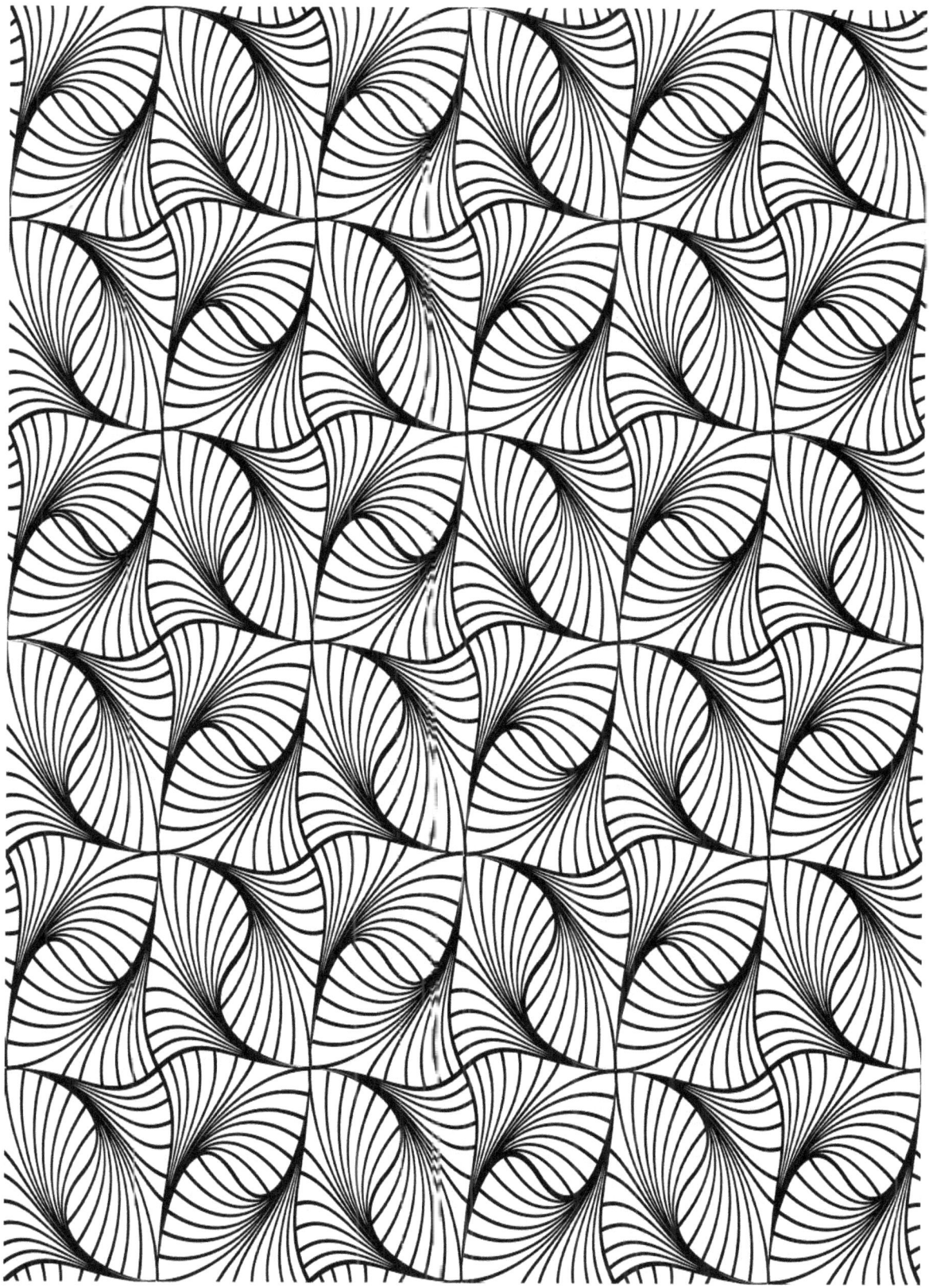

"Only I can change my life. No one can do it for me."

Carol Burnett

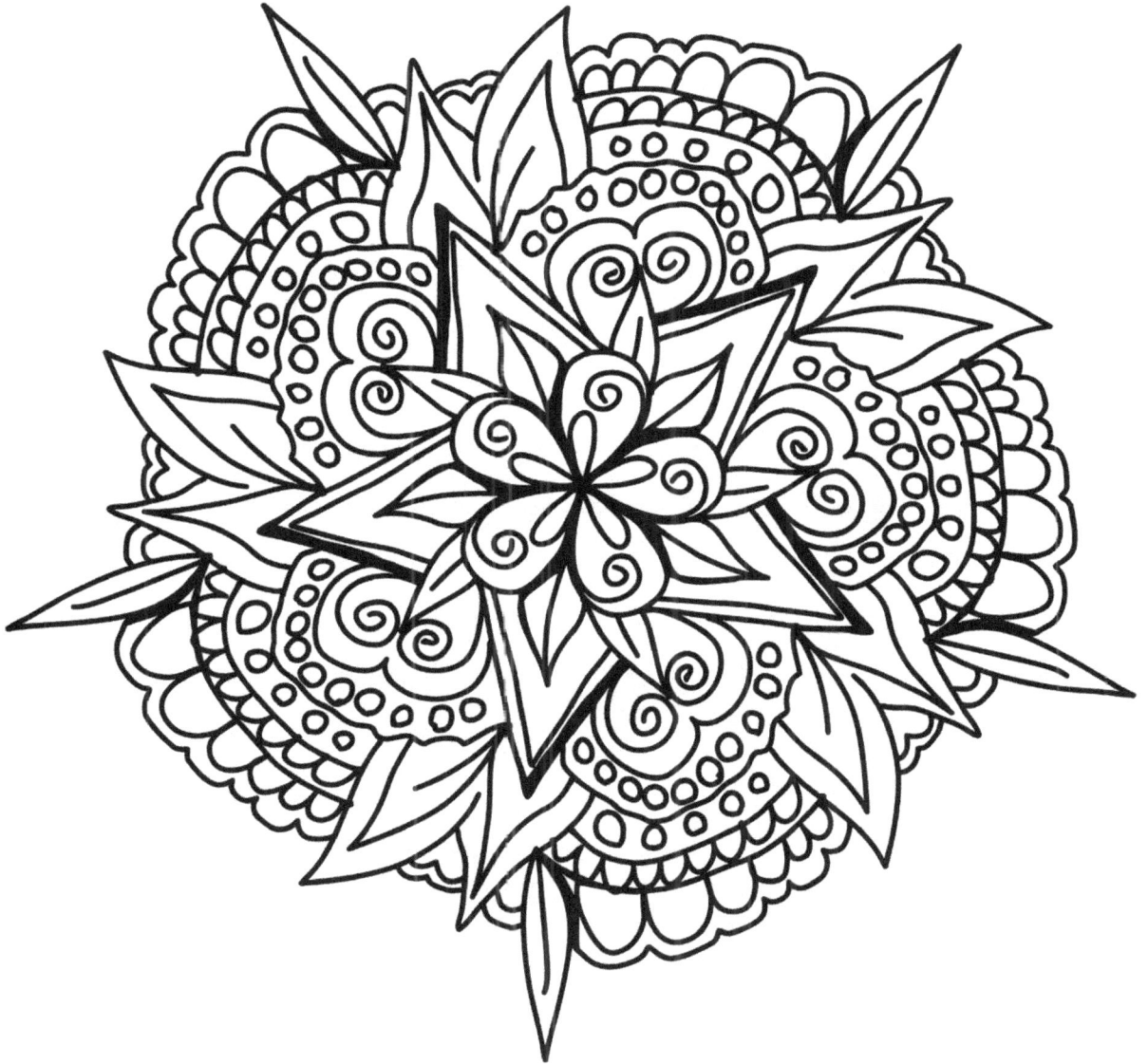

"Life is 10% what happens to you and 90% how you react to it."

Charles R. Swindoll

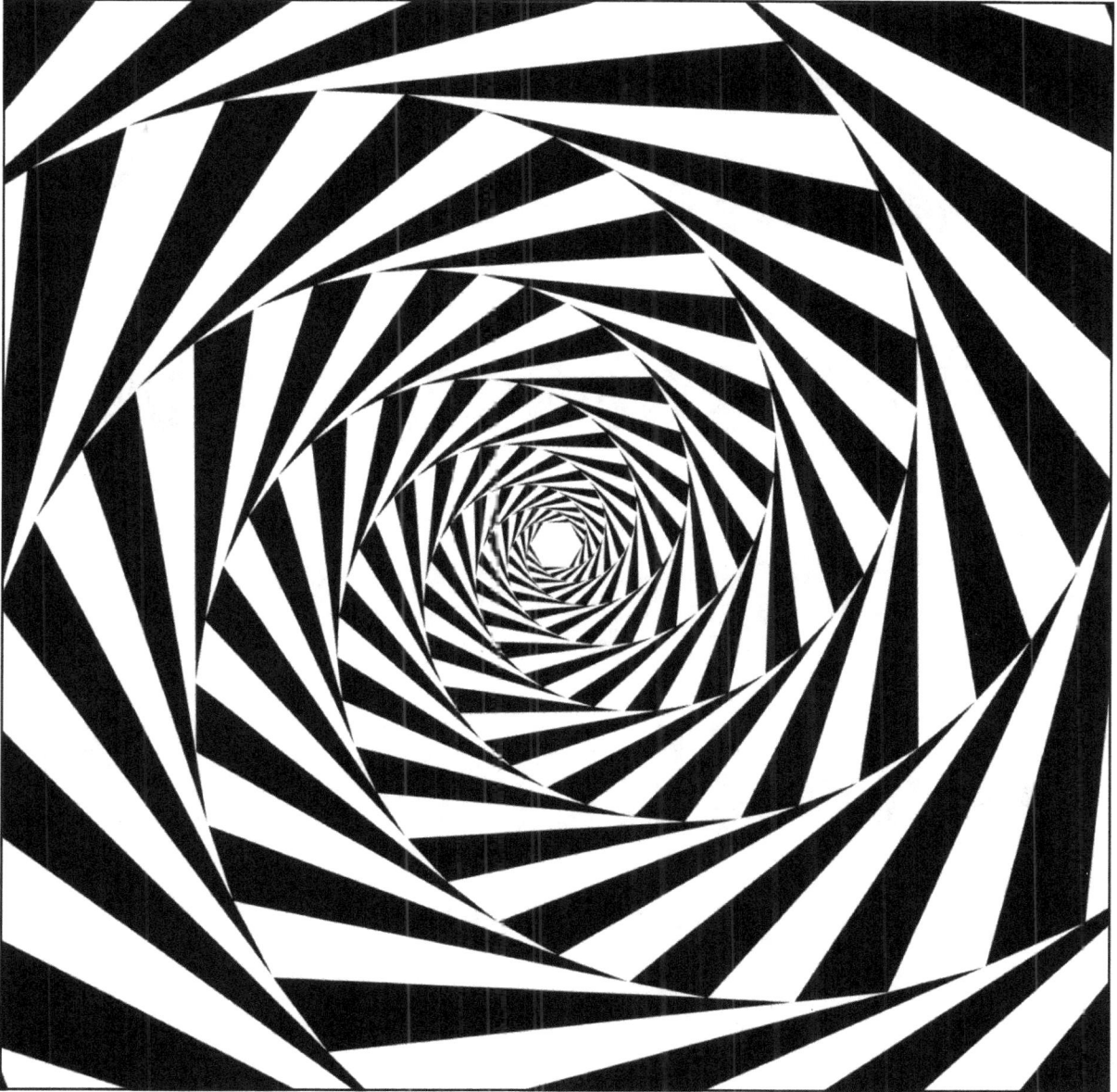

"With the new day comes new strength and new thoughts."

Eleanor Roosevelt

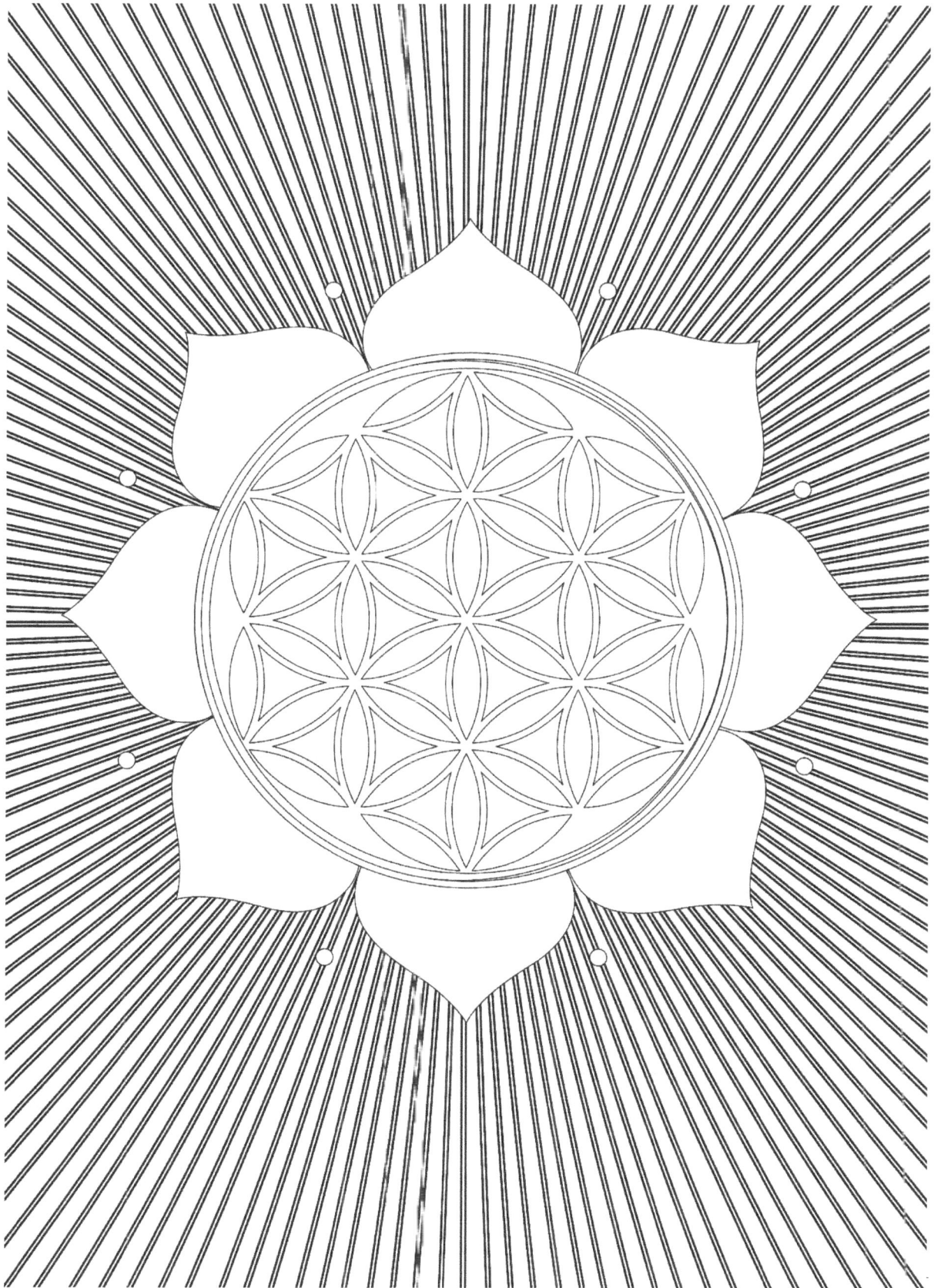

"It always seems impossible until it's done."

Nelson Mandela

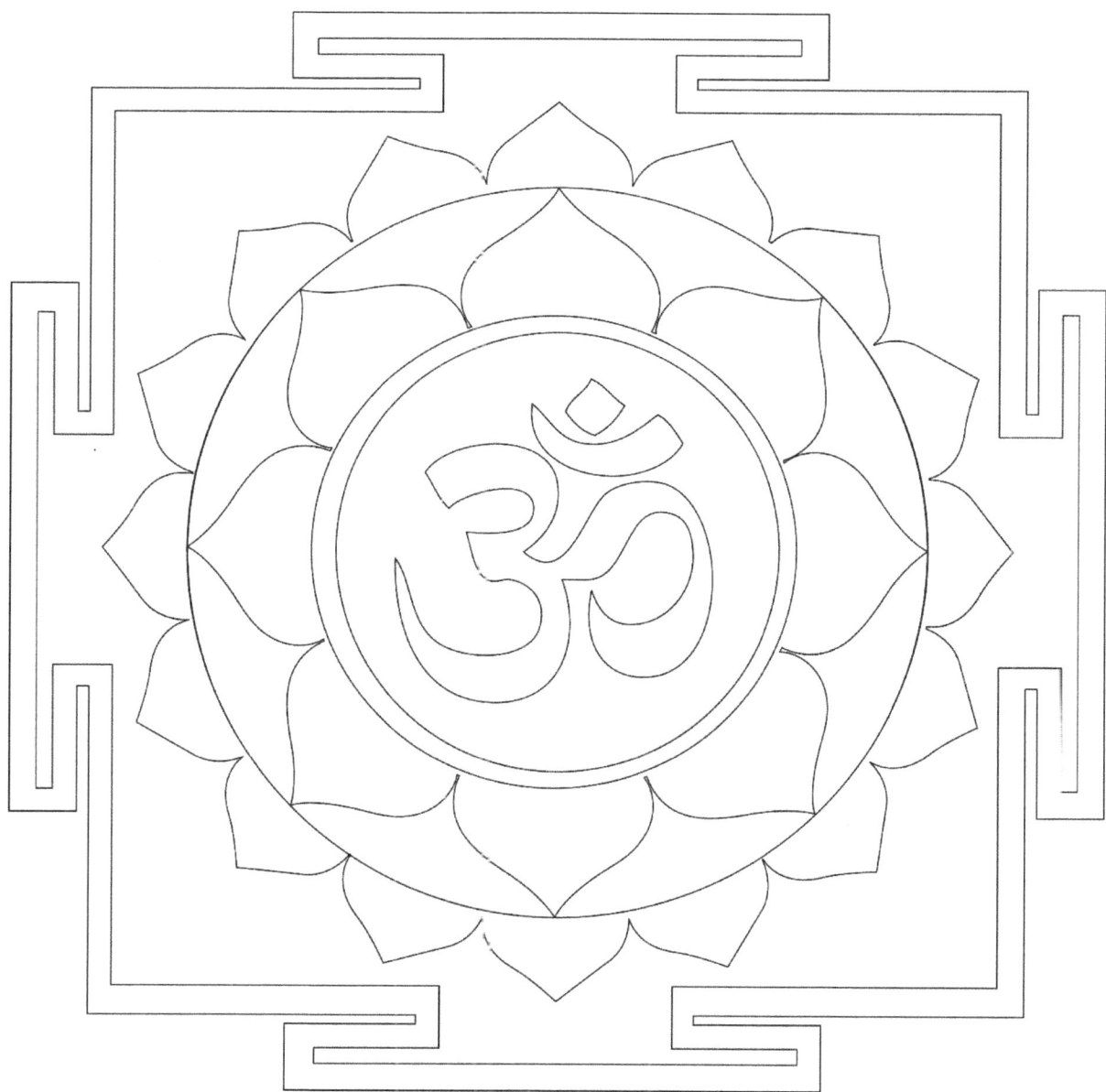

"Our greatest weakness lies in giving up. The most certain way to succeed is always to try just one more time."

Thomas A. Edison

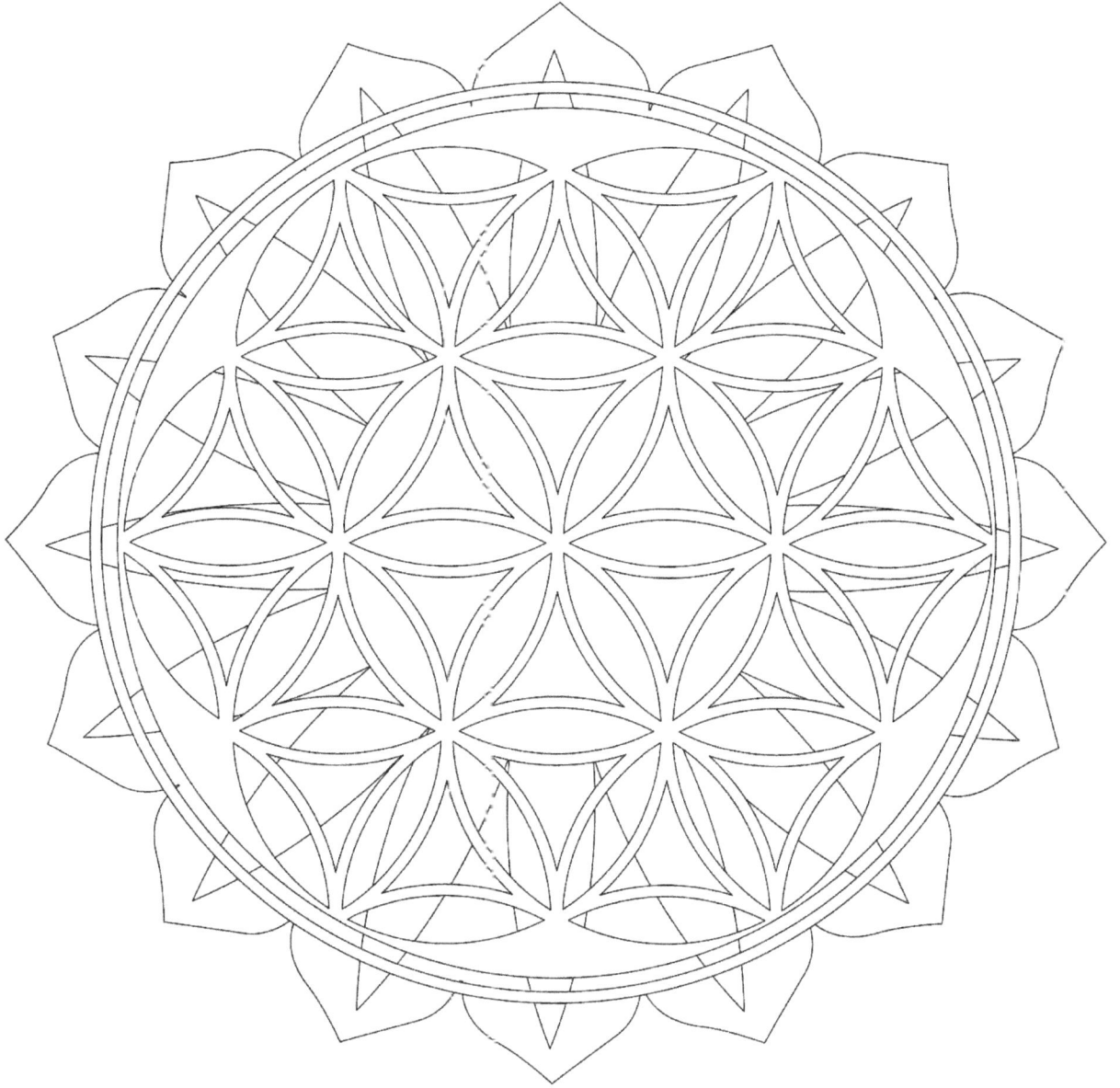

"You will never win if you never begin."

Helen Rowland

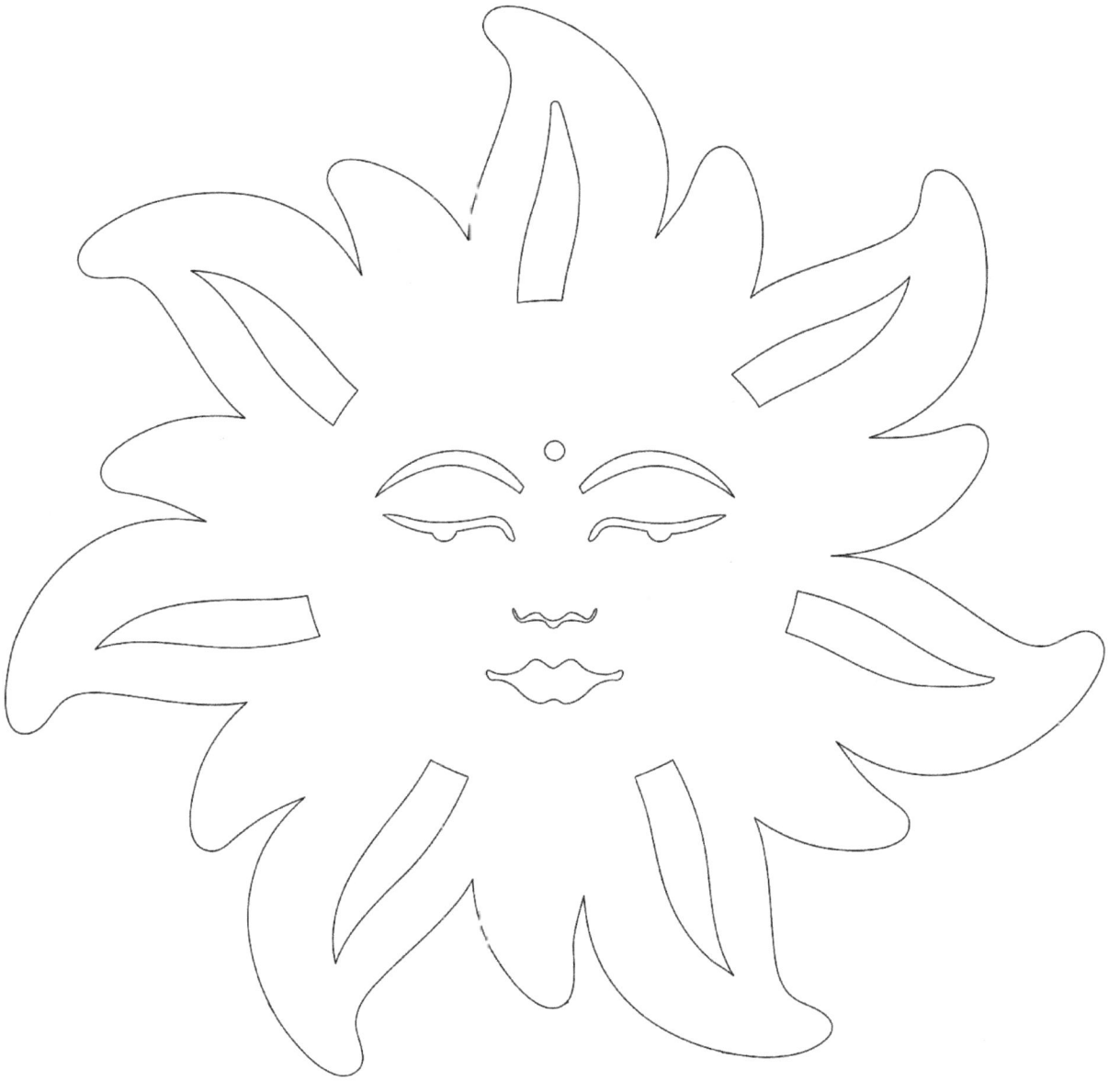

"Visualize this thing that you want, see it, feel it, believe in it. Make your mental blue print, and begin to build."

Robert Collier

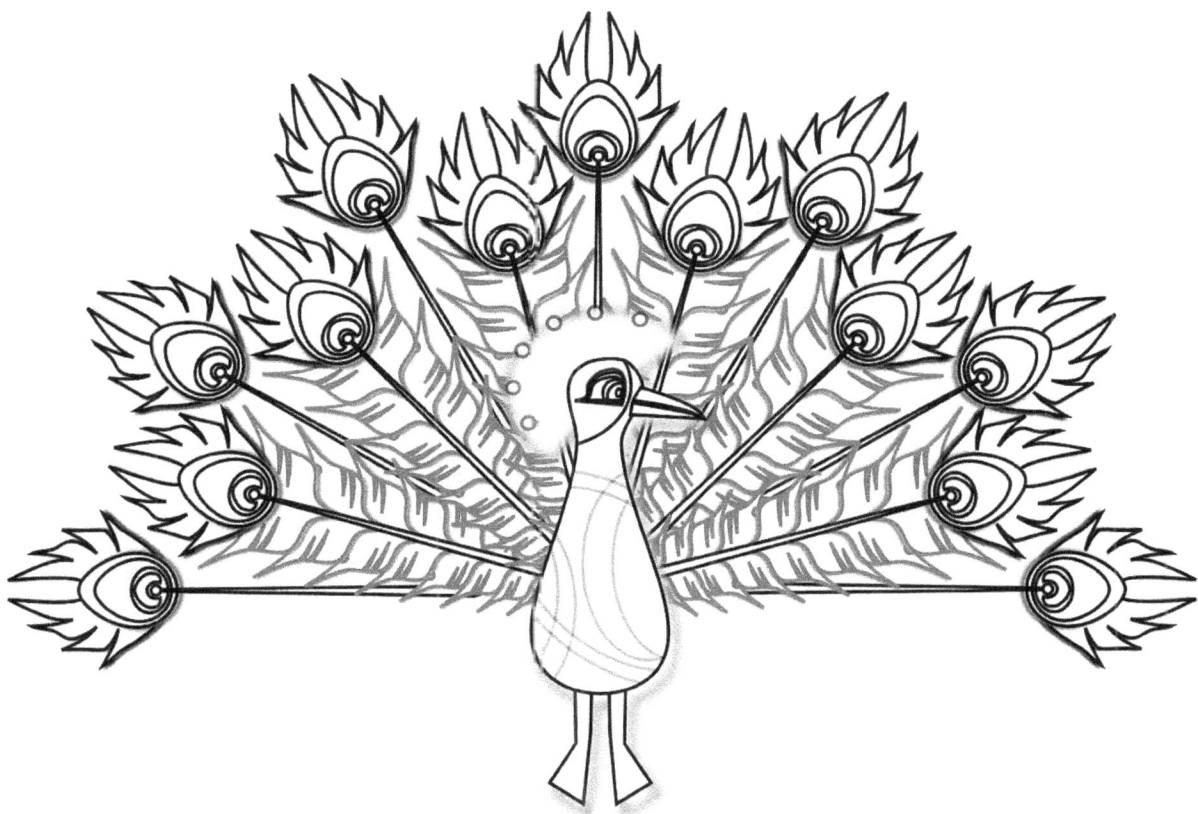

"When you confront a problem, you begin to solve it."

Rudy Giuliani

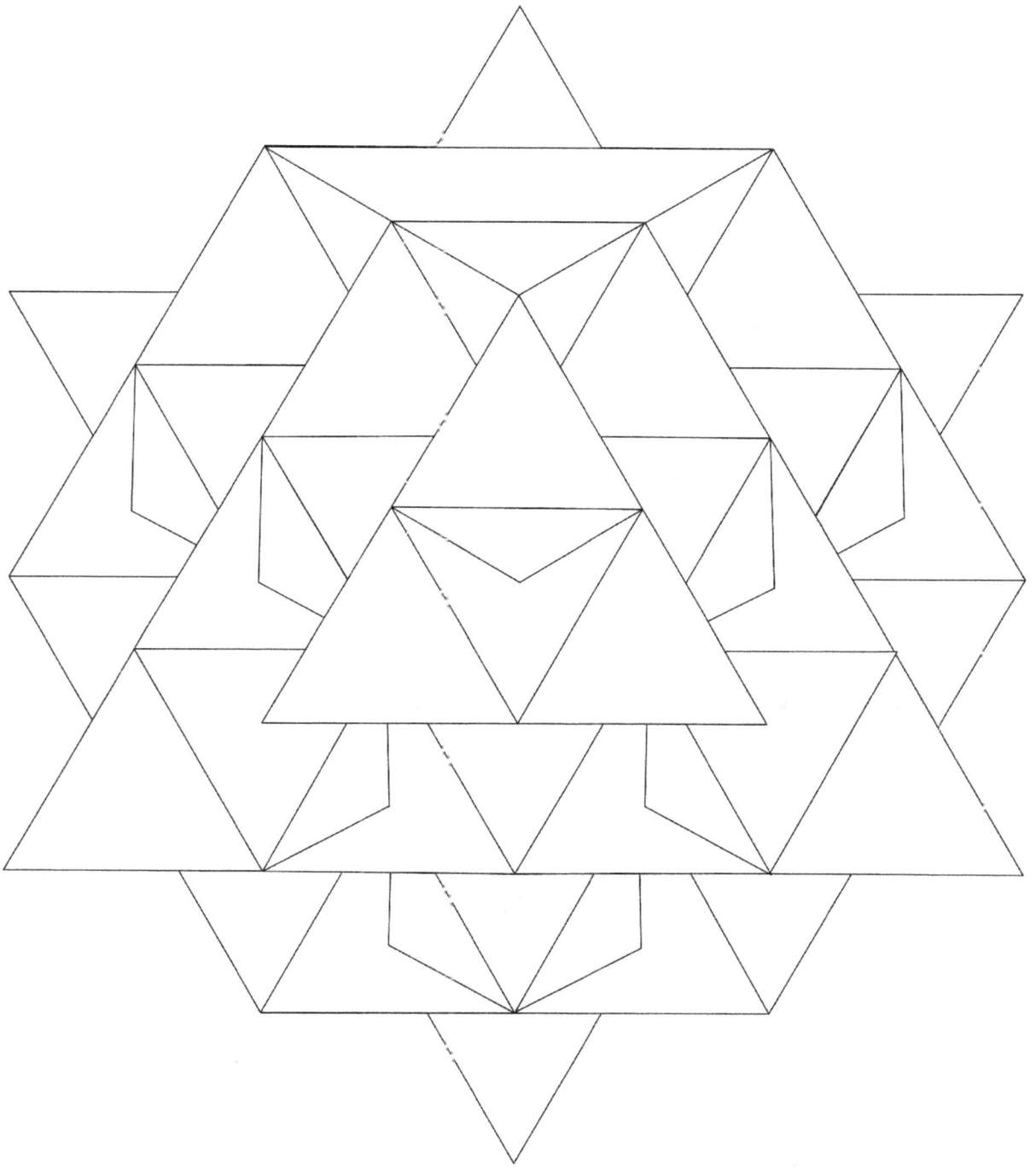

"The starting point of all achievement is desire."

Napolean Hill

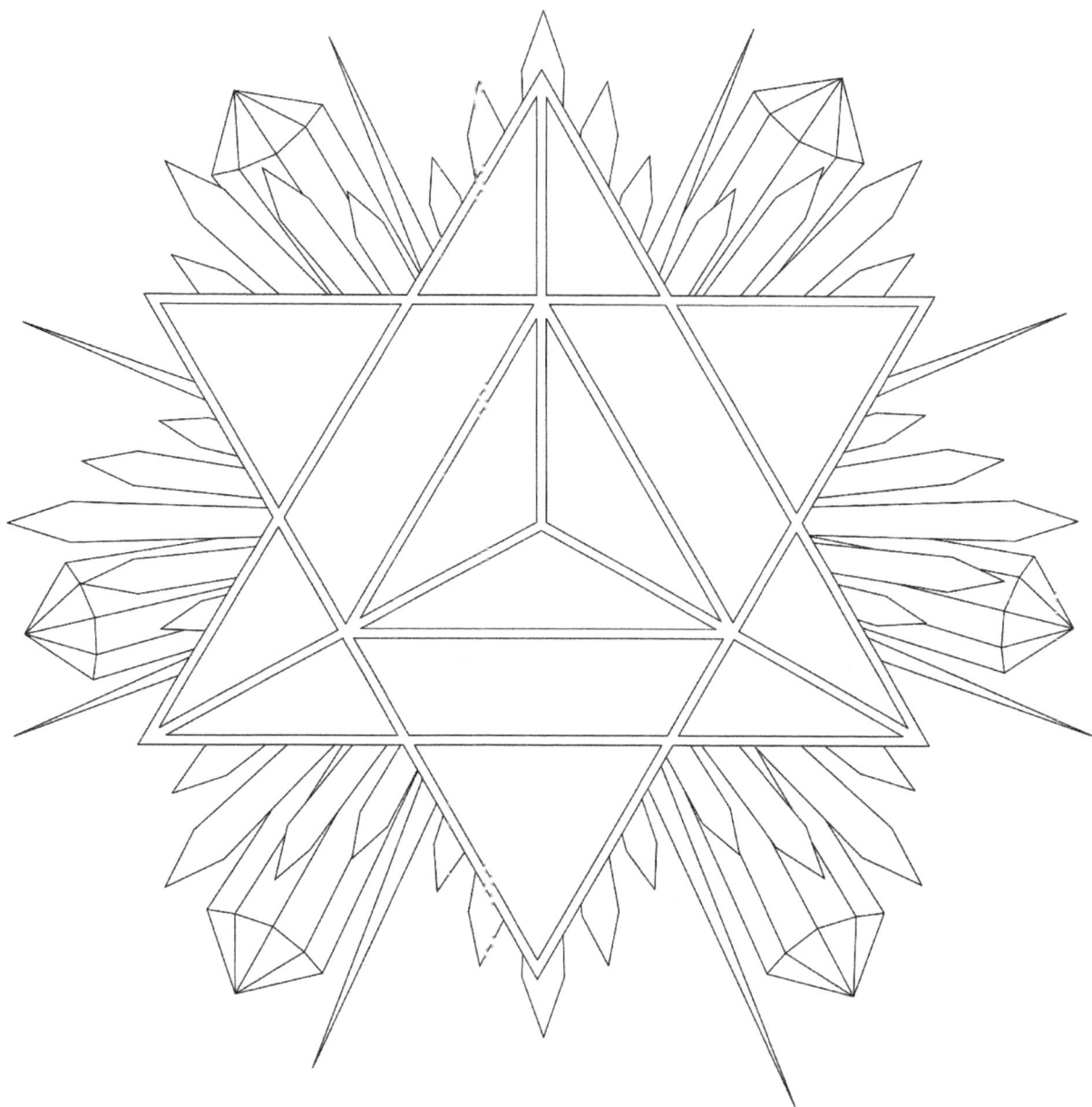

"Success is liking yourself, liking what you do, and liking how you do it."

Maya Angelou

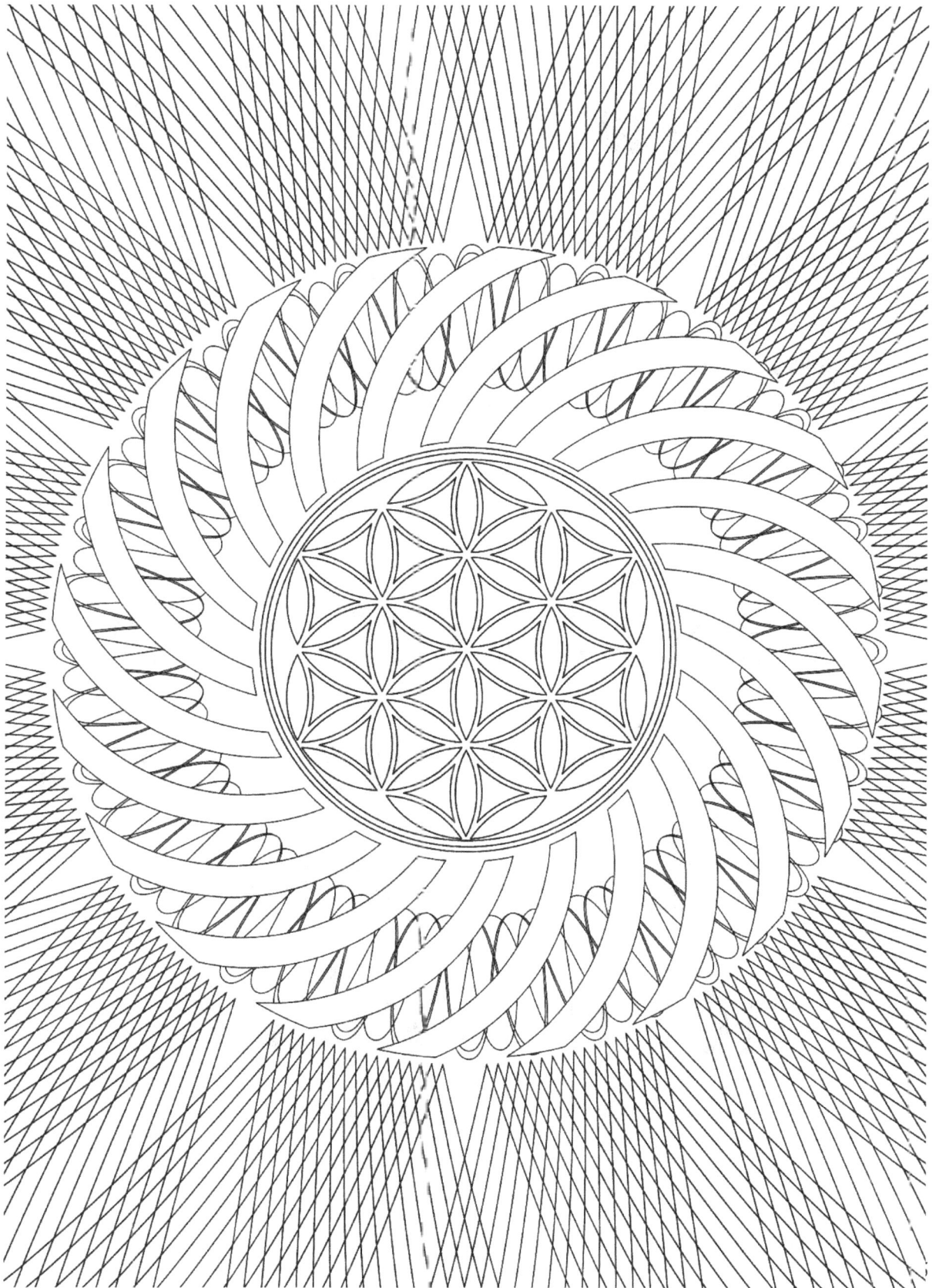

"You measure the size of the accomplishment by the obstacles you had to overcome to reach your goals."

Booker T. Washington

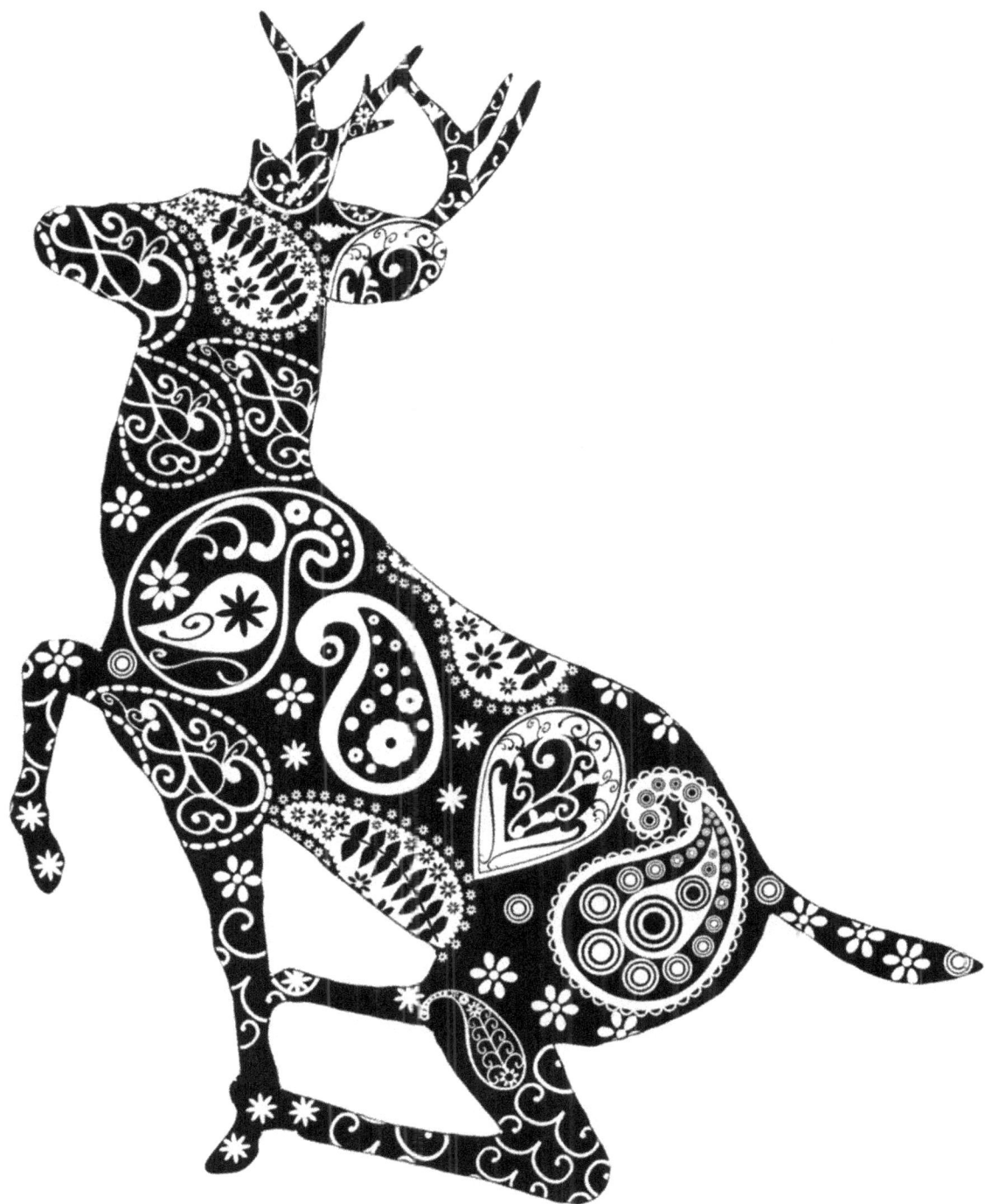

"Every great story on the planet happened when someone decided not to give up, but kept going no matter what."

Spryte Loriano

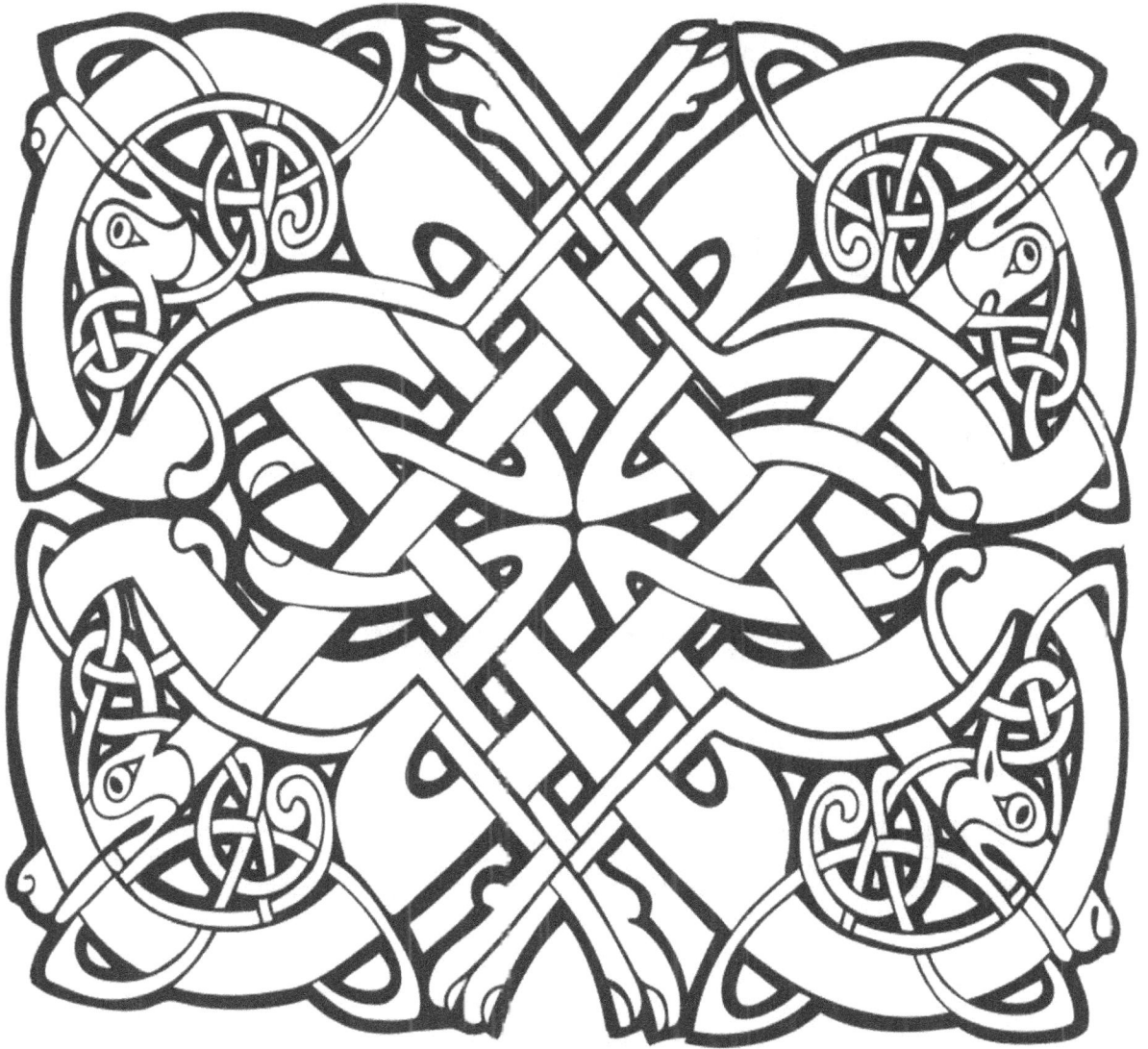

"Hardships often prepare ordinary people for an extraordinary destiny."

C.S. Lewis

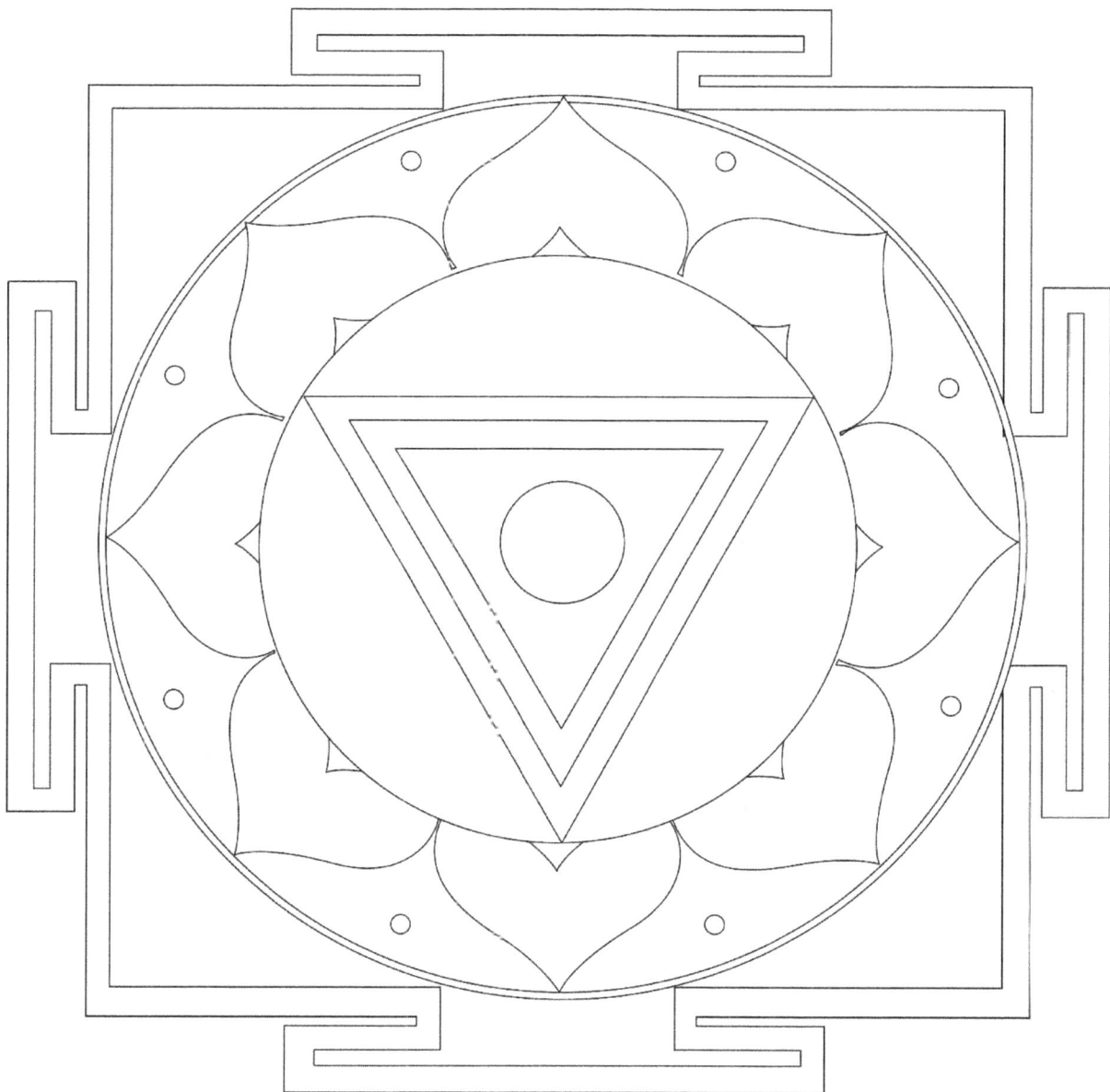

"The first step is to say you can!"

Will Smith

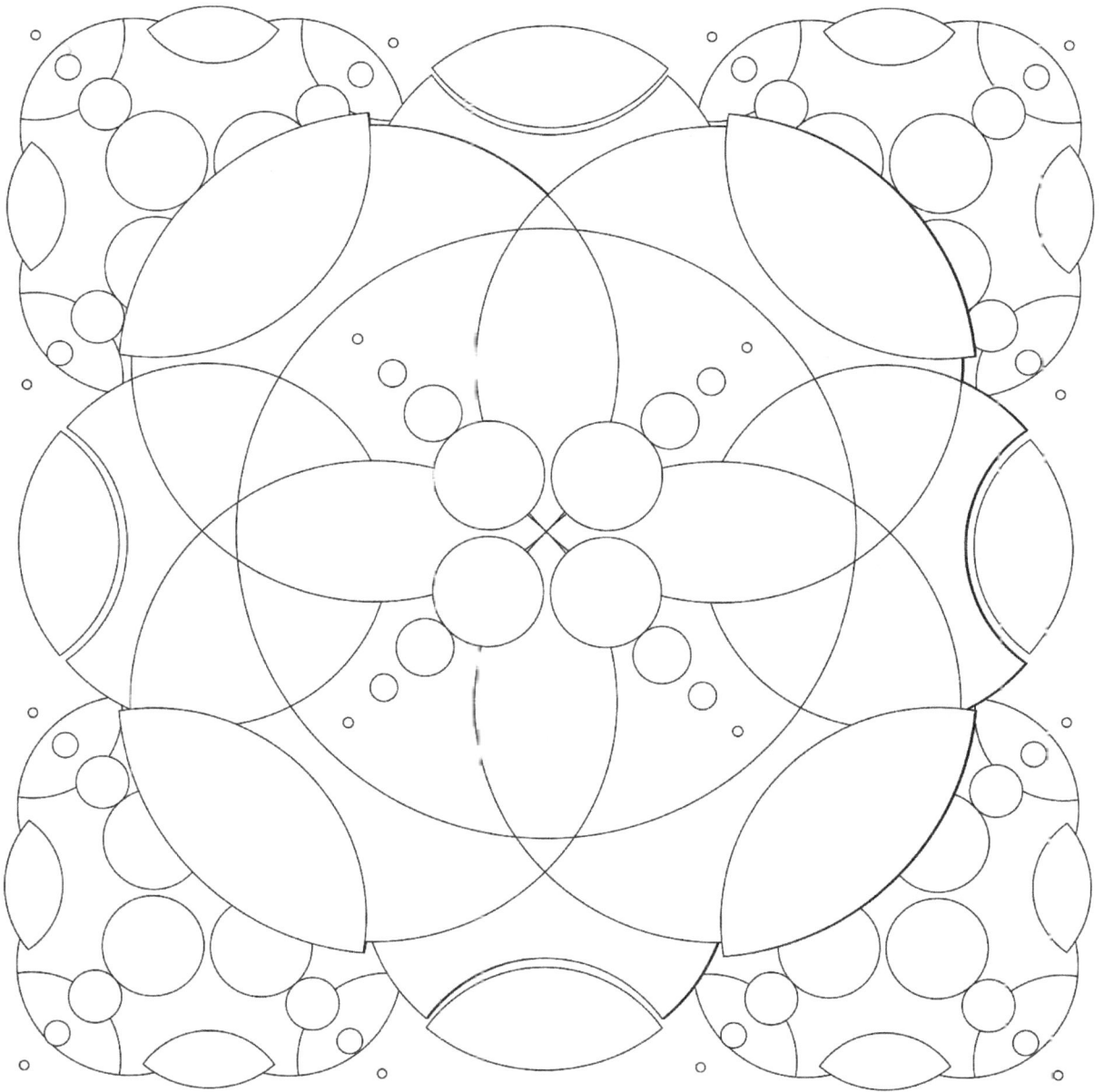

"Success is the sum of all small efforts, repeated day in and day out."

Robert Collier

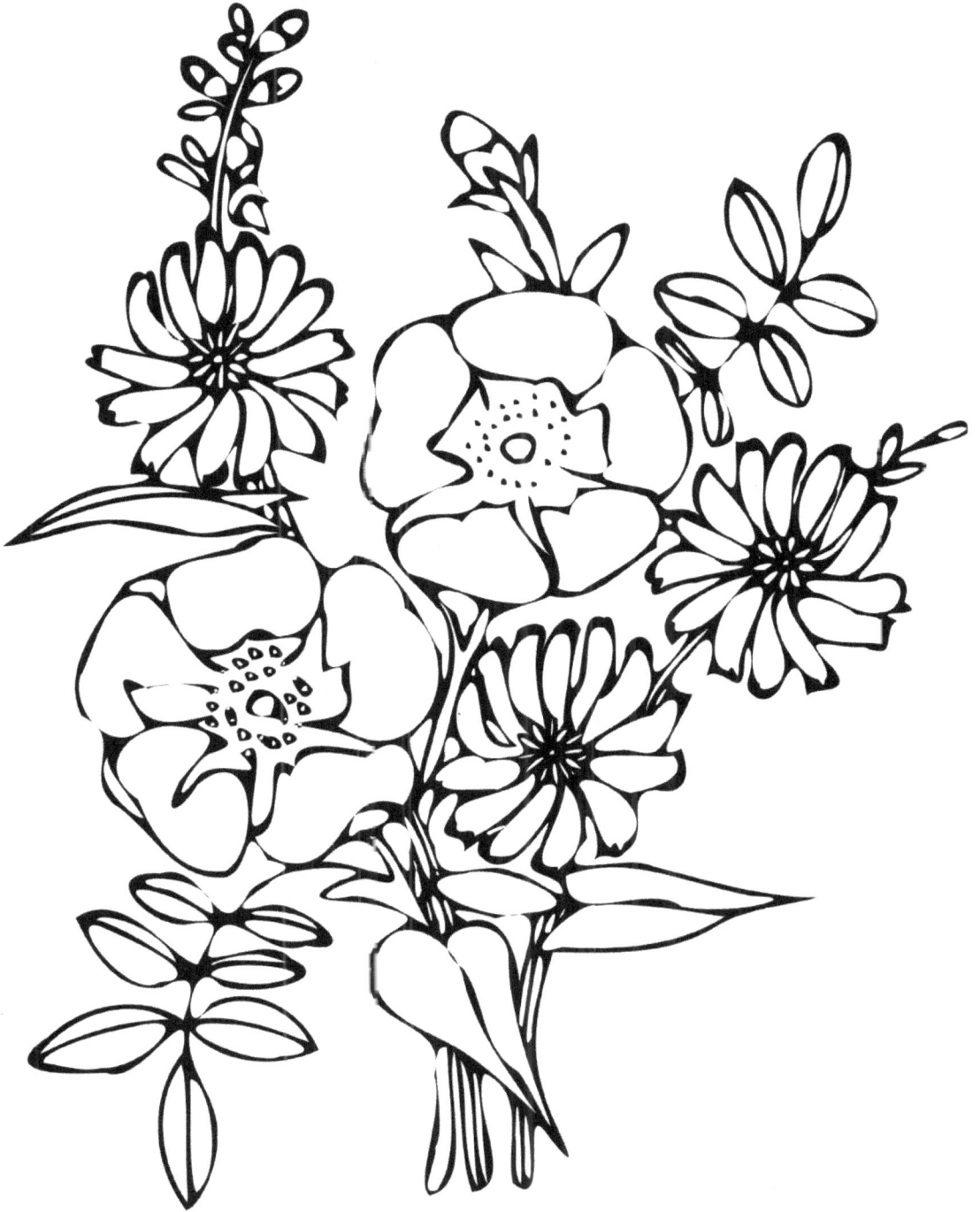

"When you adopt a positive mindset, you are harnessing the power of choice."

Victor Schueller

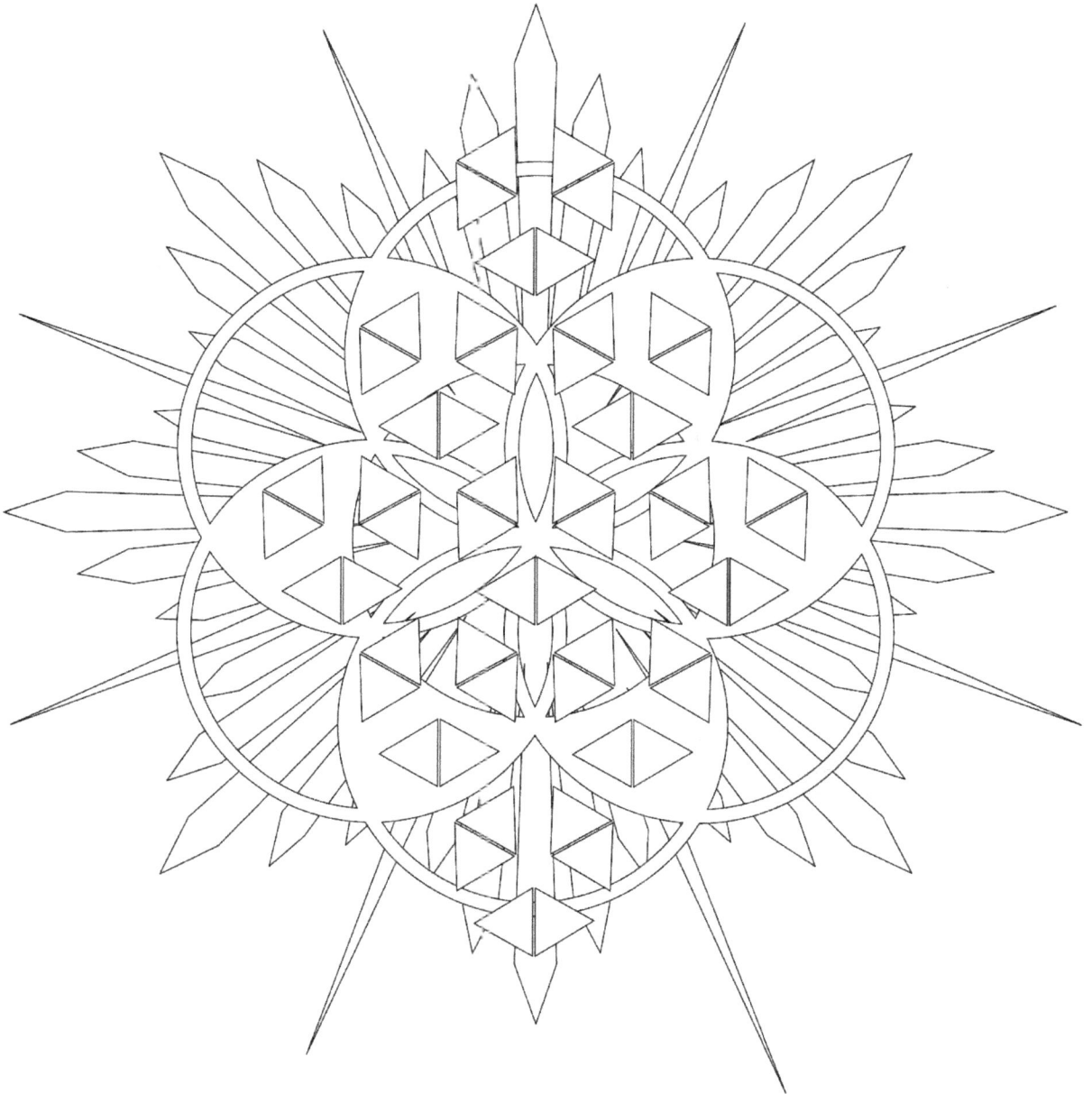

"It is often in the darkest skies that we see the brightest stars."

Richard Evans

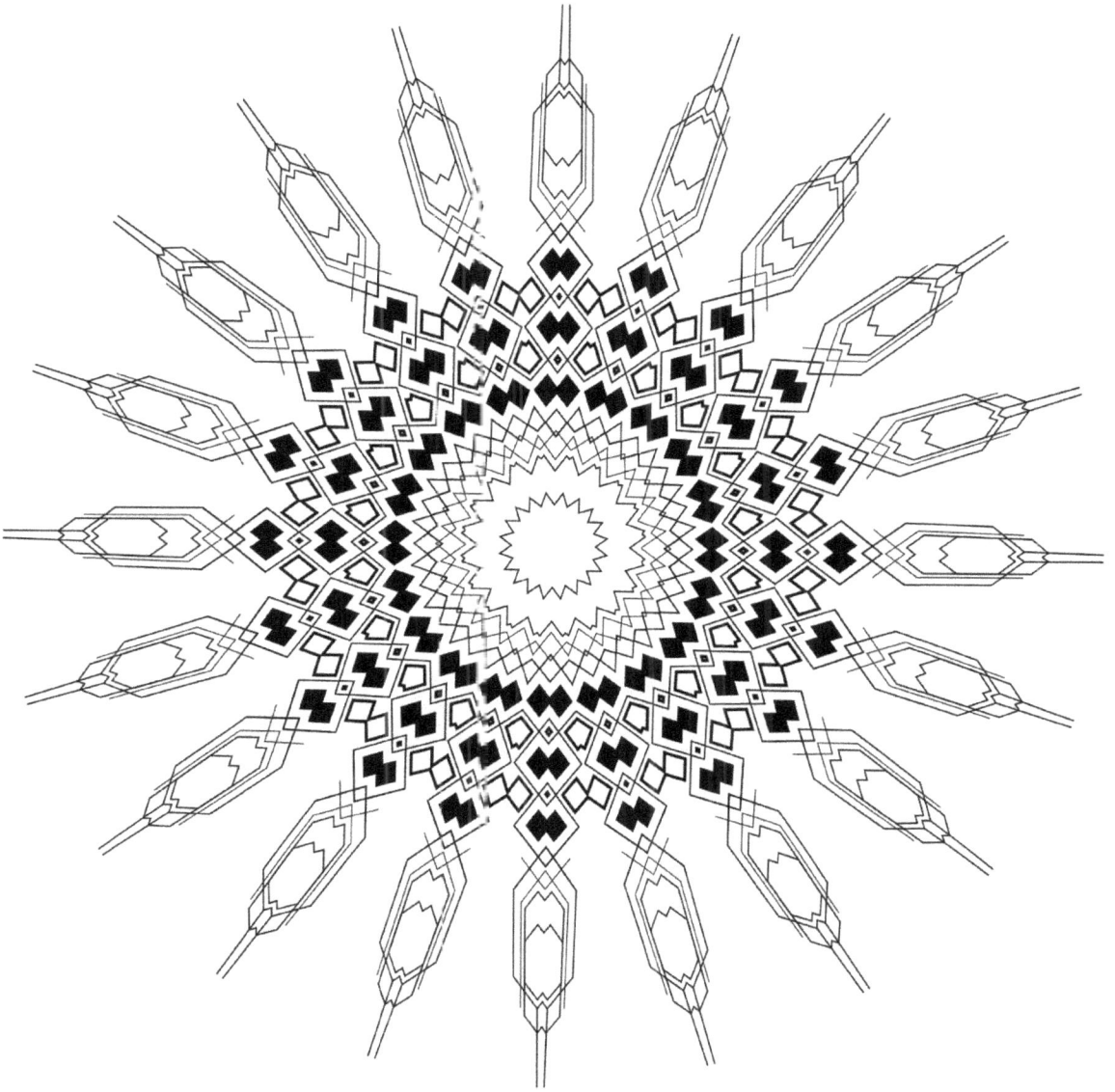

"A negative mind will never give you a positive life."

Zig Ziglar

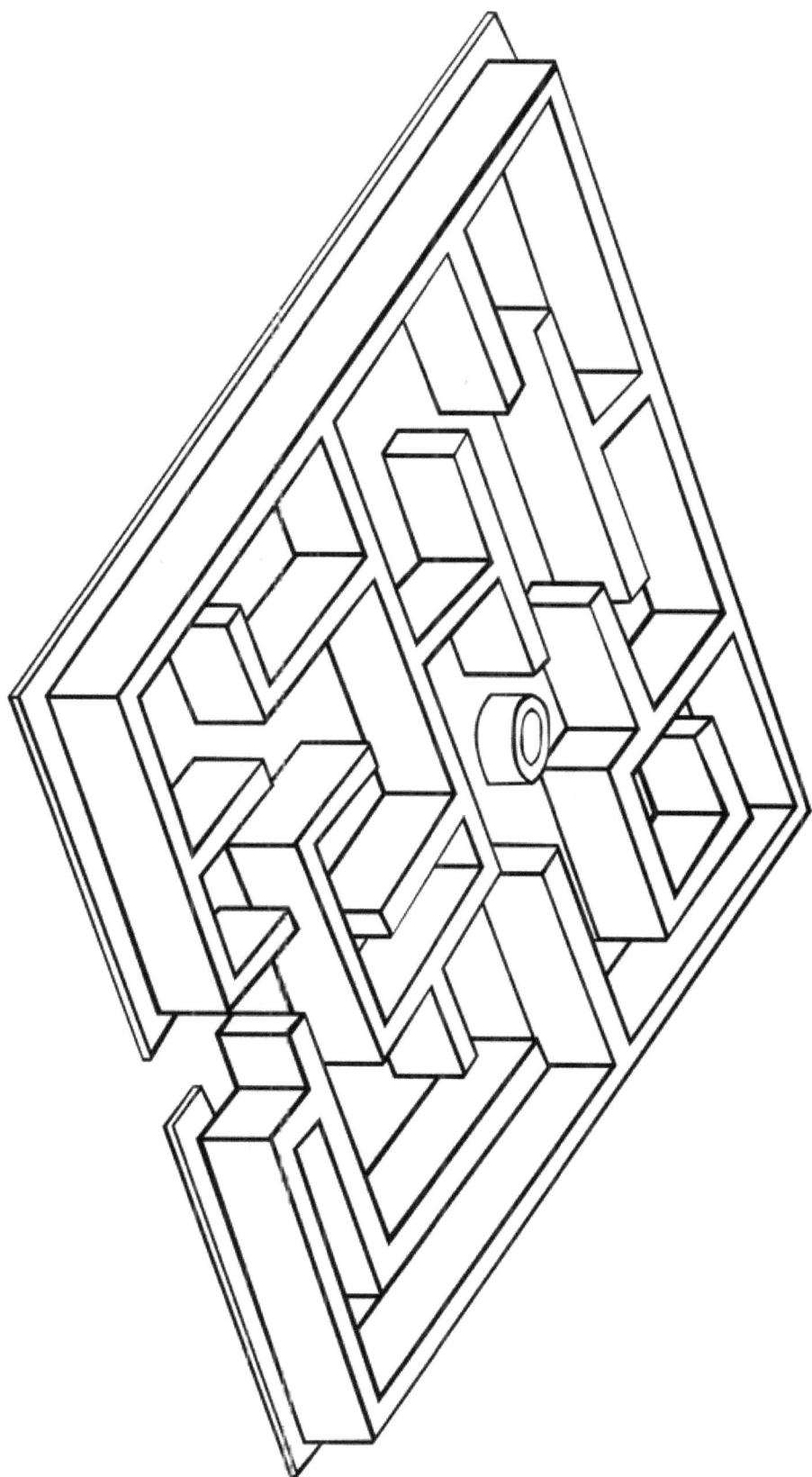

"If you can quit for a day, you can quit for a lifetime."

Benjamin Alire Saenz

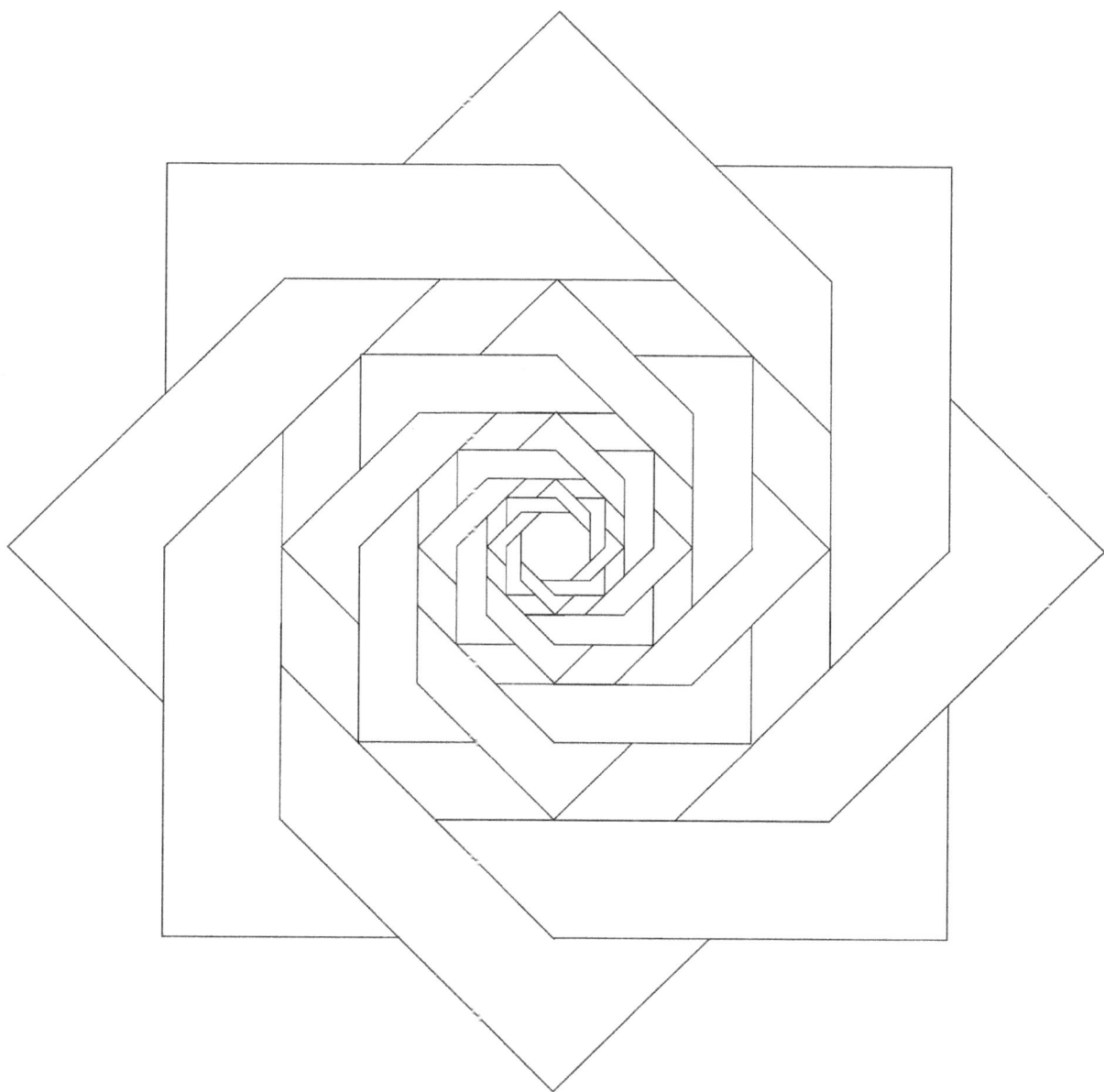

"Hardships often prepare ordinary people for an extraordinary destiny."

C.S. Lewis

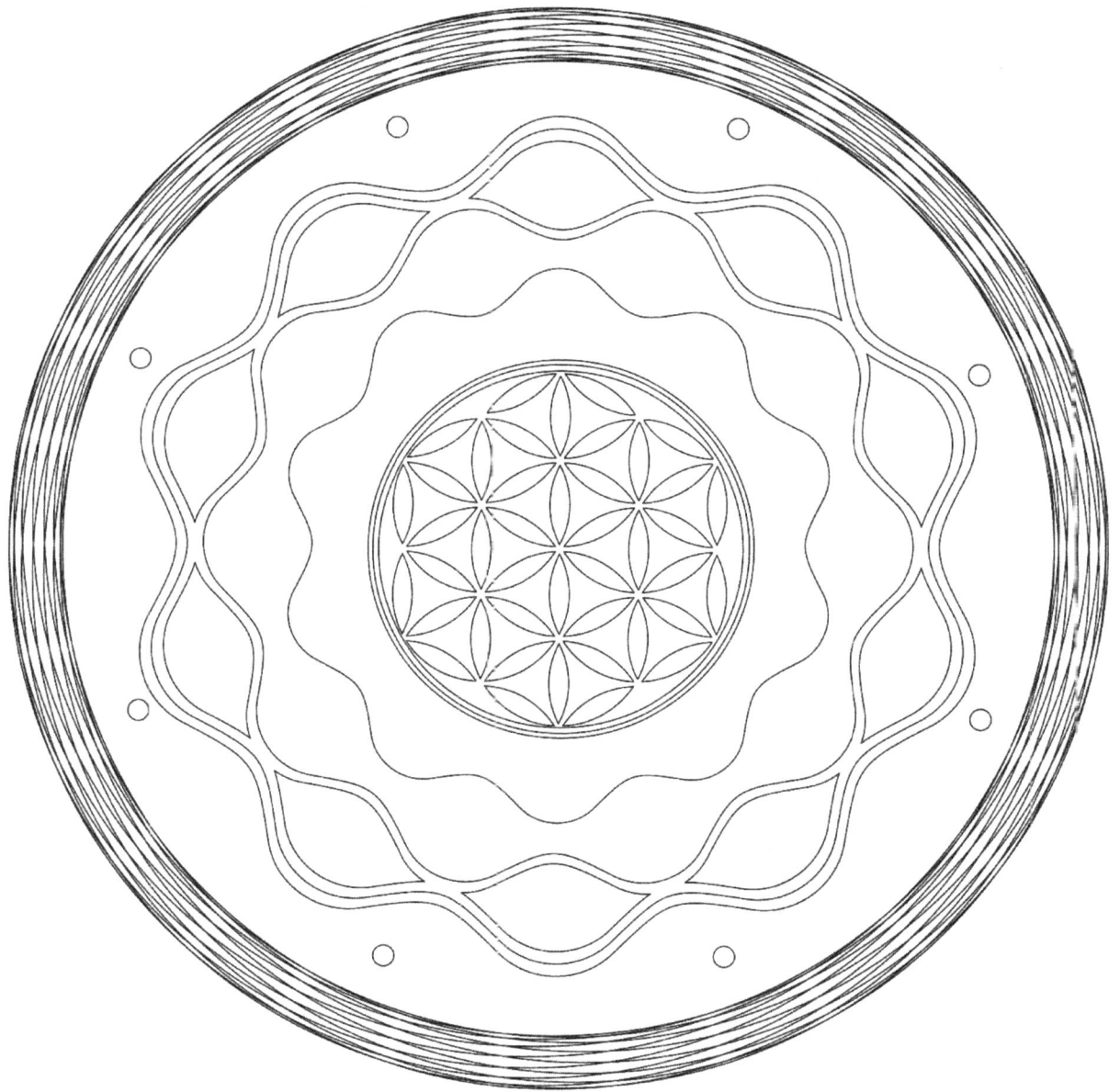

"When everything seems to be going against you, remember that the airplane takes off against the wind, not with it."

Henry Ford

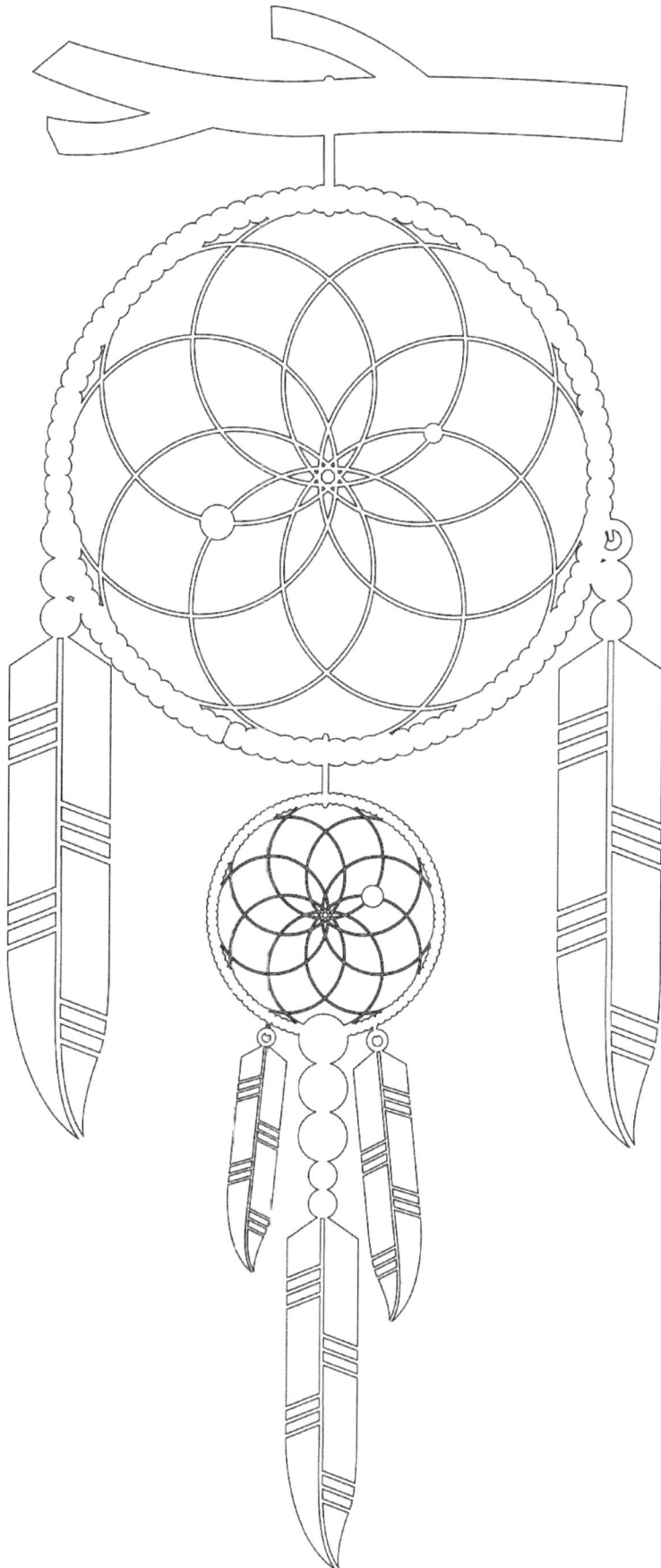

"Our greatest glory is not in never failing, but in rising up every time we fail."

Ralph Waldo Emerson

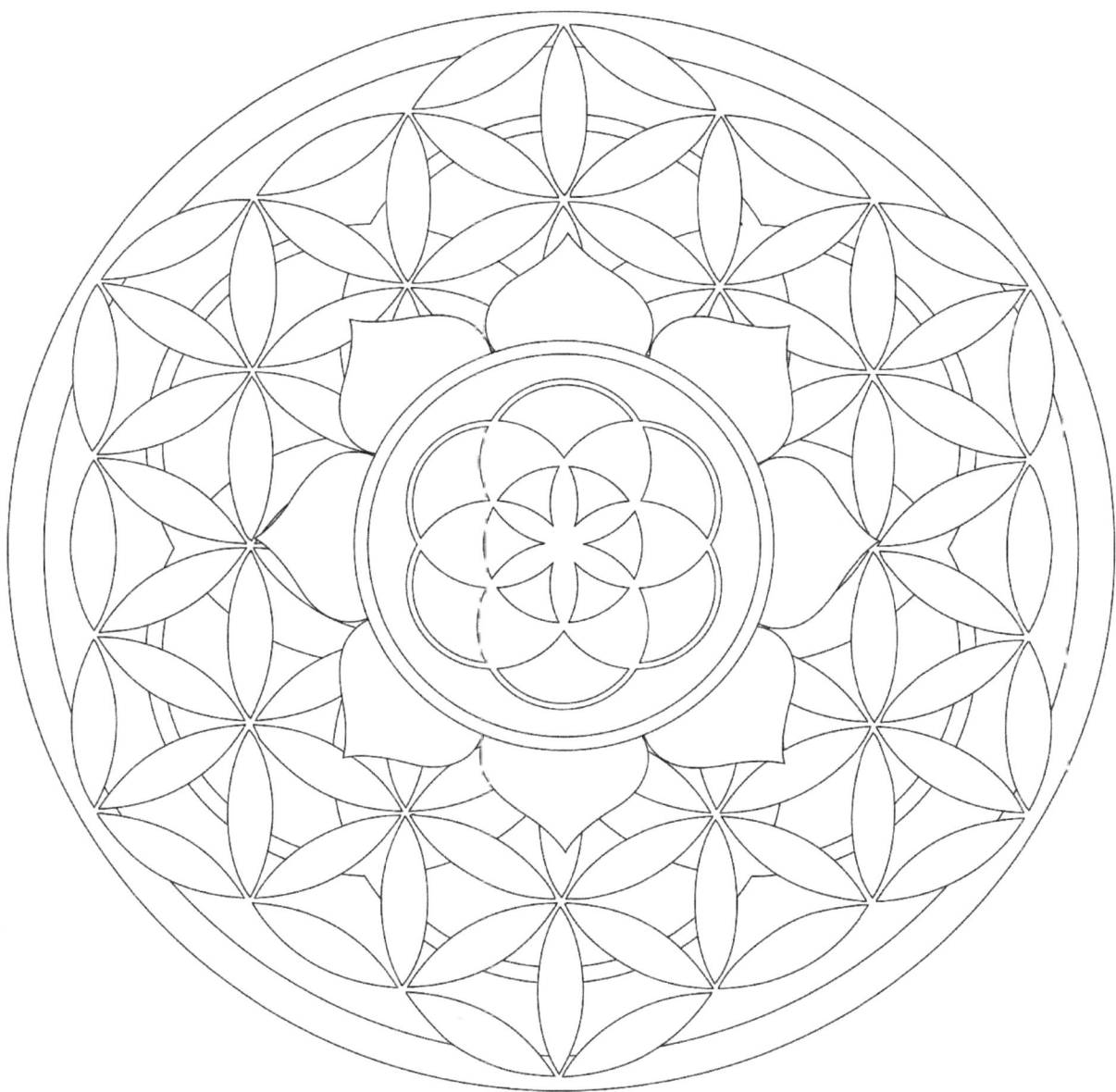

"It always seems impossible until it's done."

Nelson Mandela

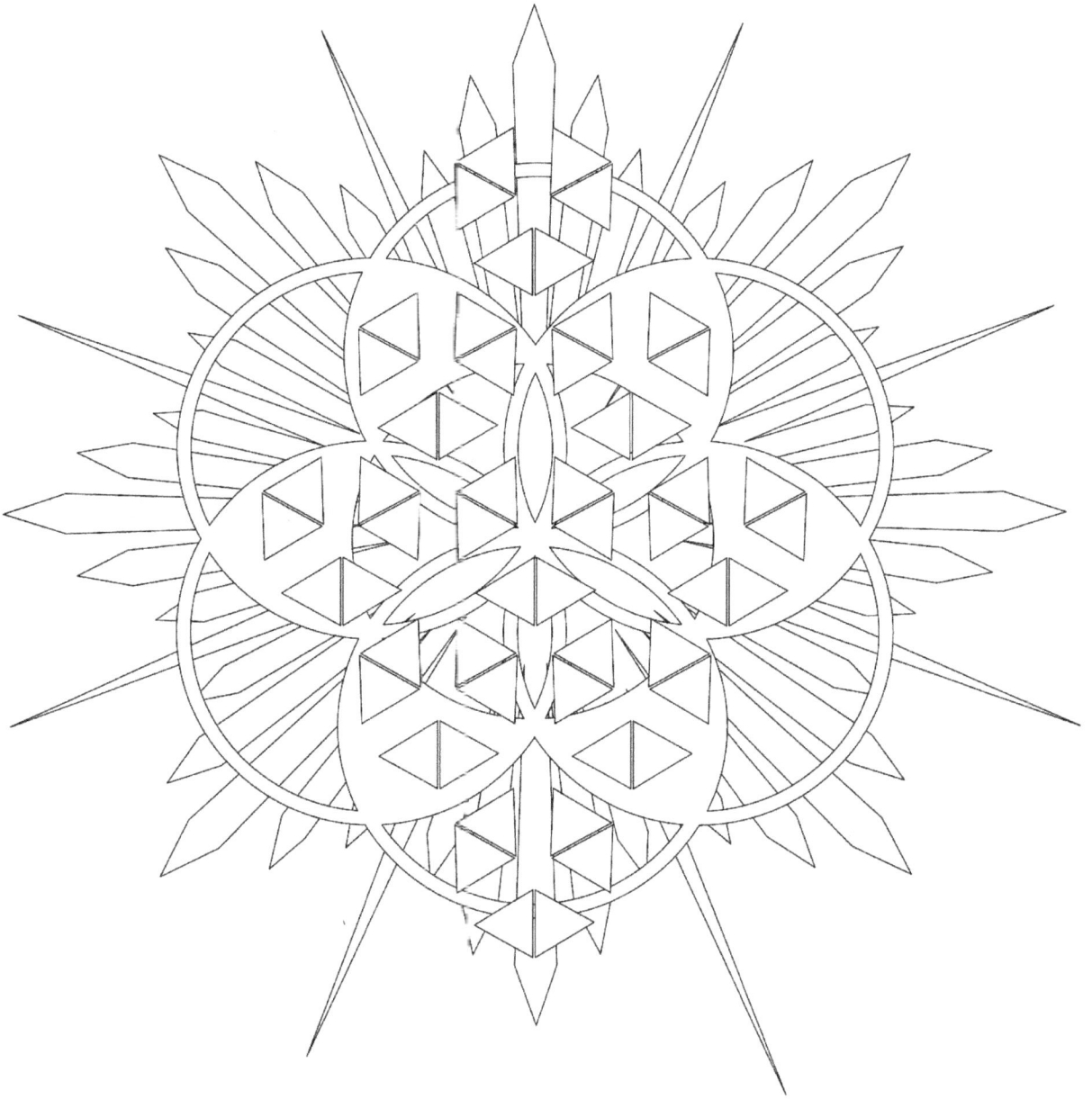

"Even the darkest night will end, and the sun will rise."

Victor Hugo

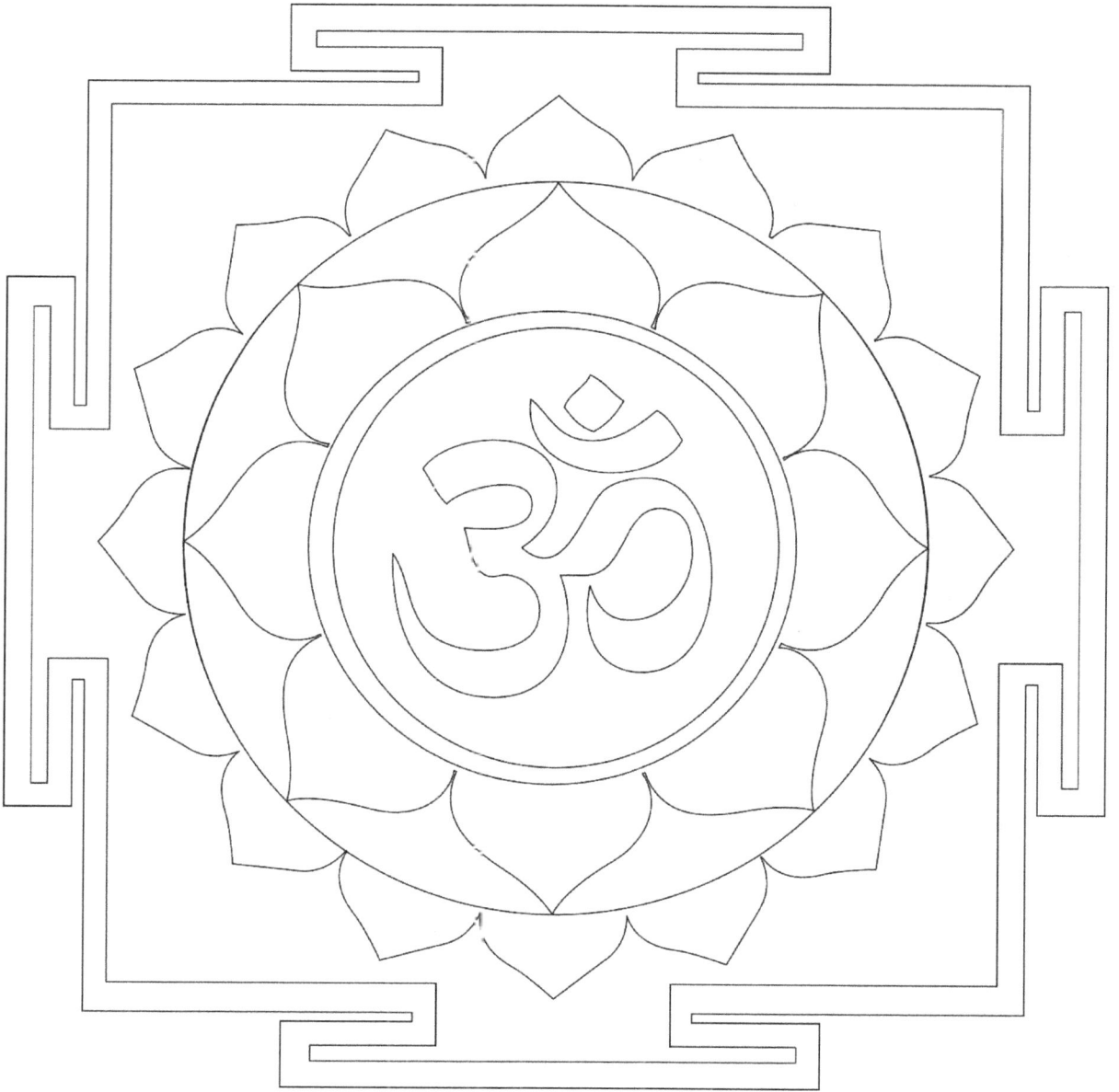

"Don't let the past steal your present."

Terri Guillemets

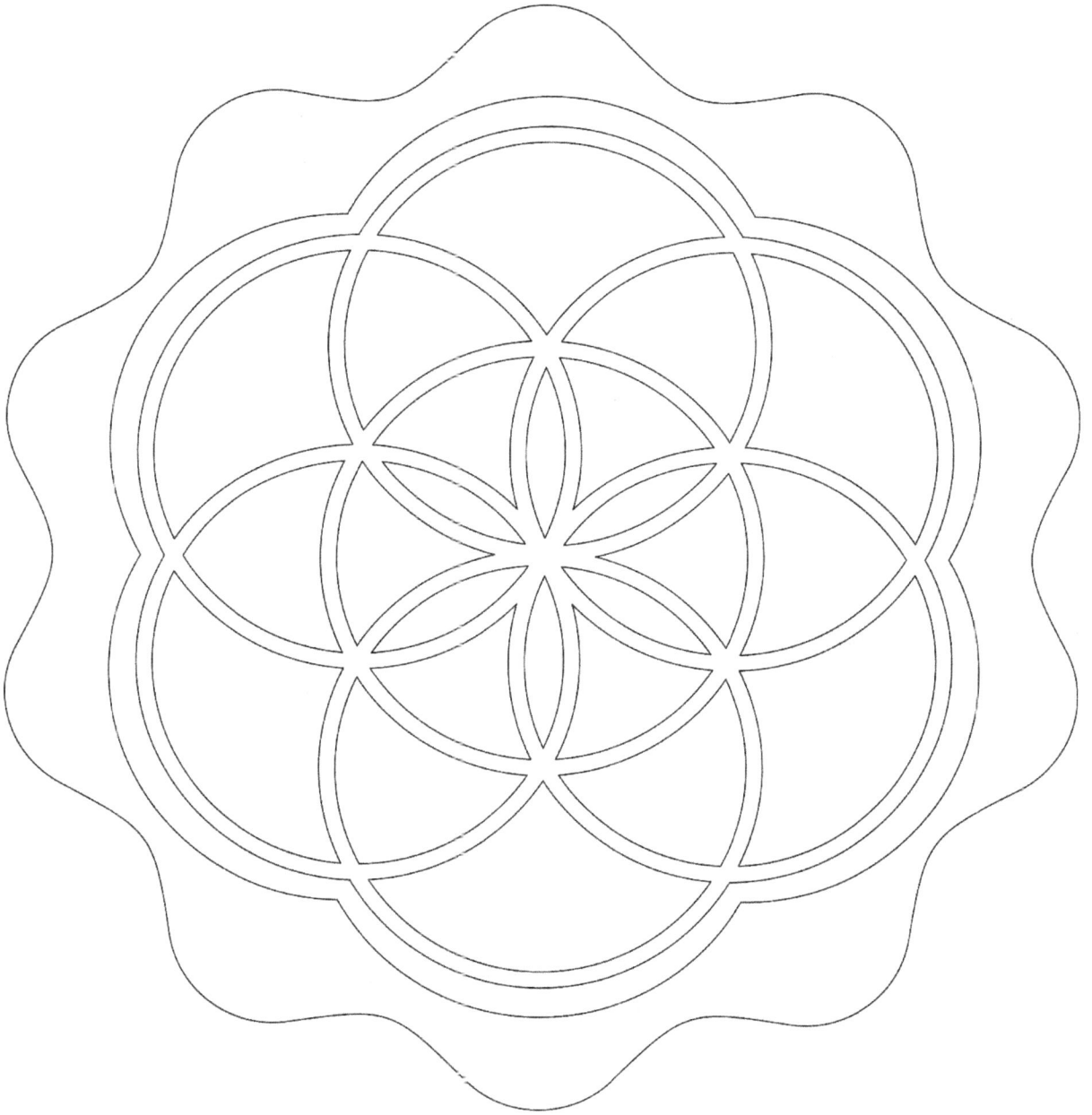

"Taking responsibility for your beliefs and judgments gives you the power to change them."

Byron Katie

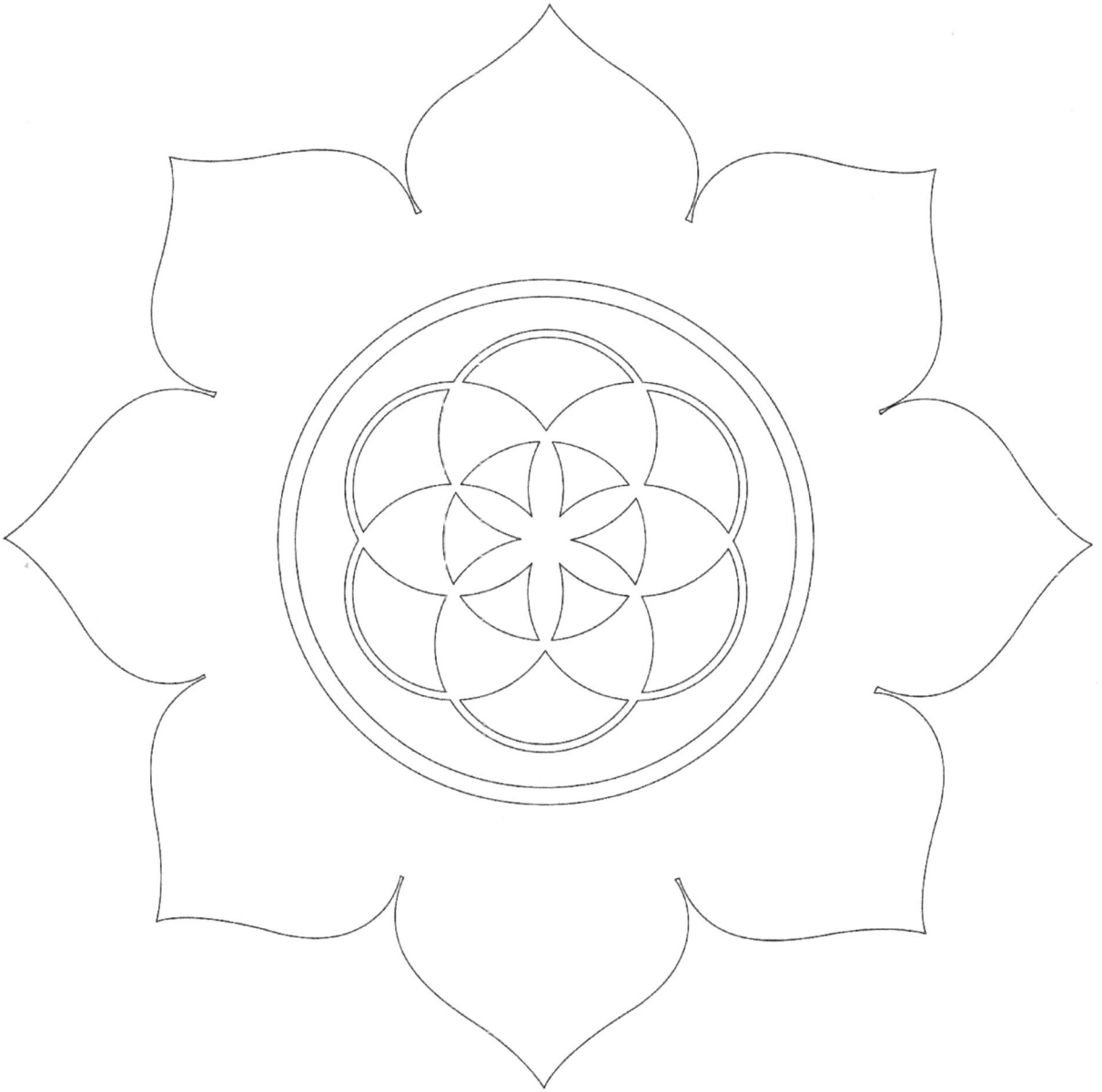

"Don't let the past steal your present."

Terri Guillemets

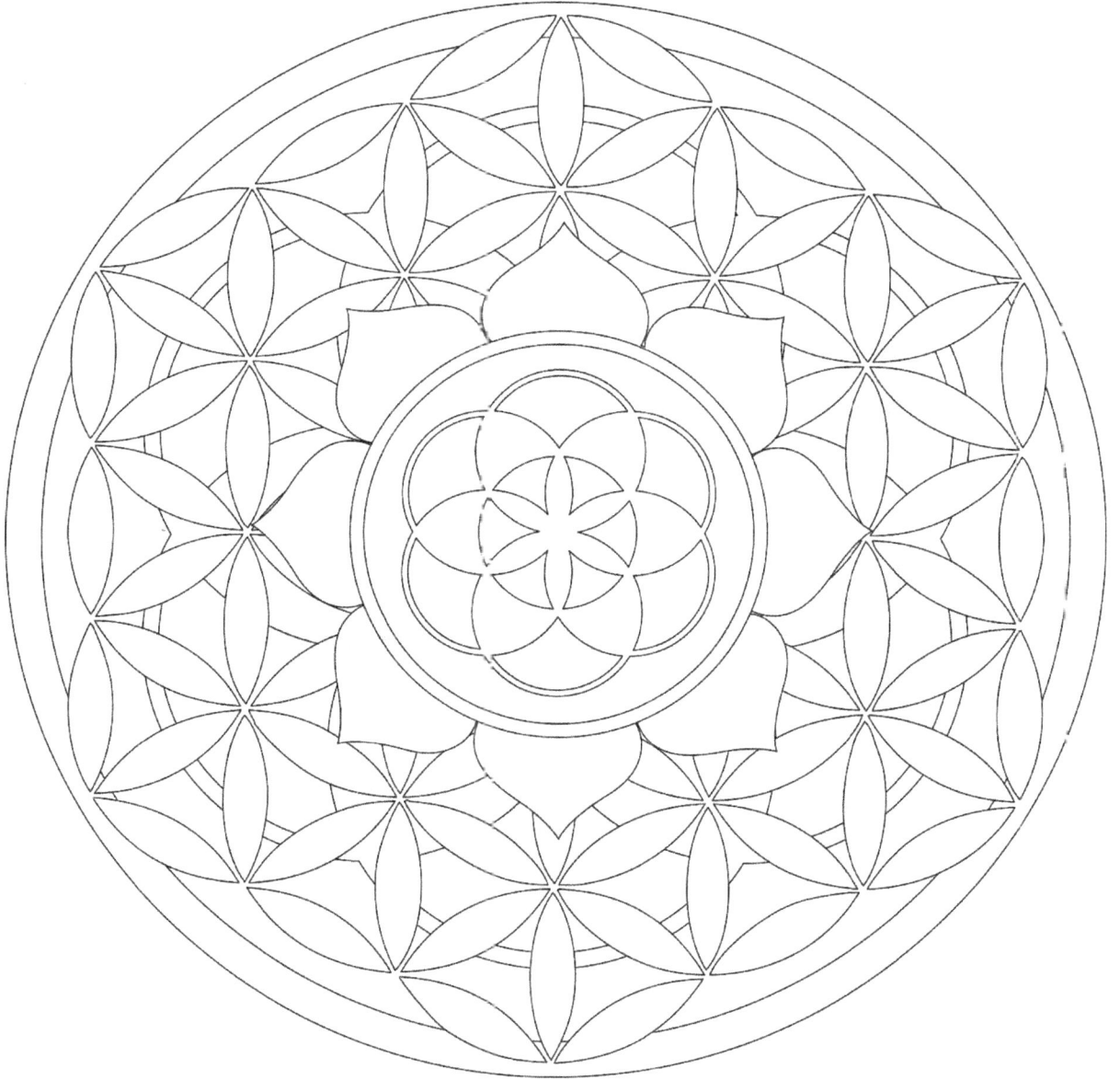

"Sometimes you can only find Heaven by slowly backing away from Hell."

Carrie Fisher

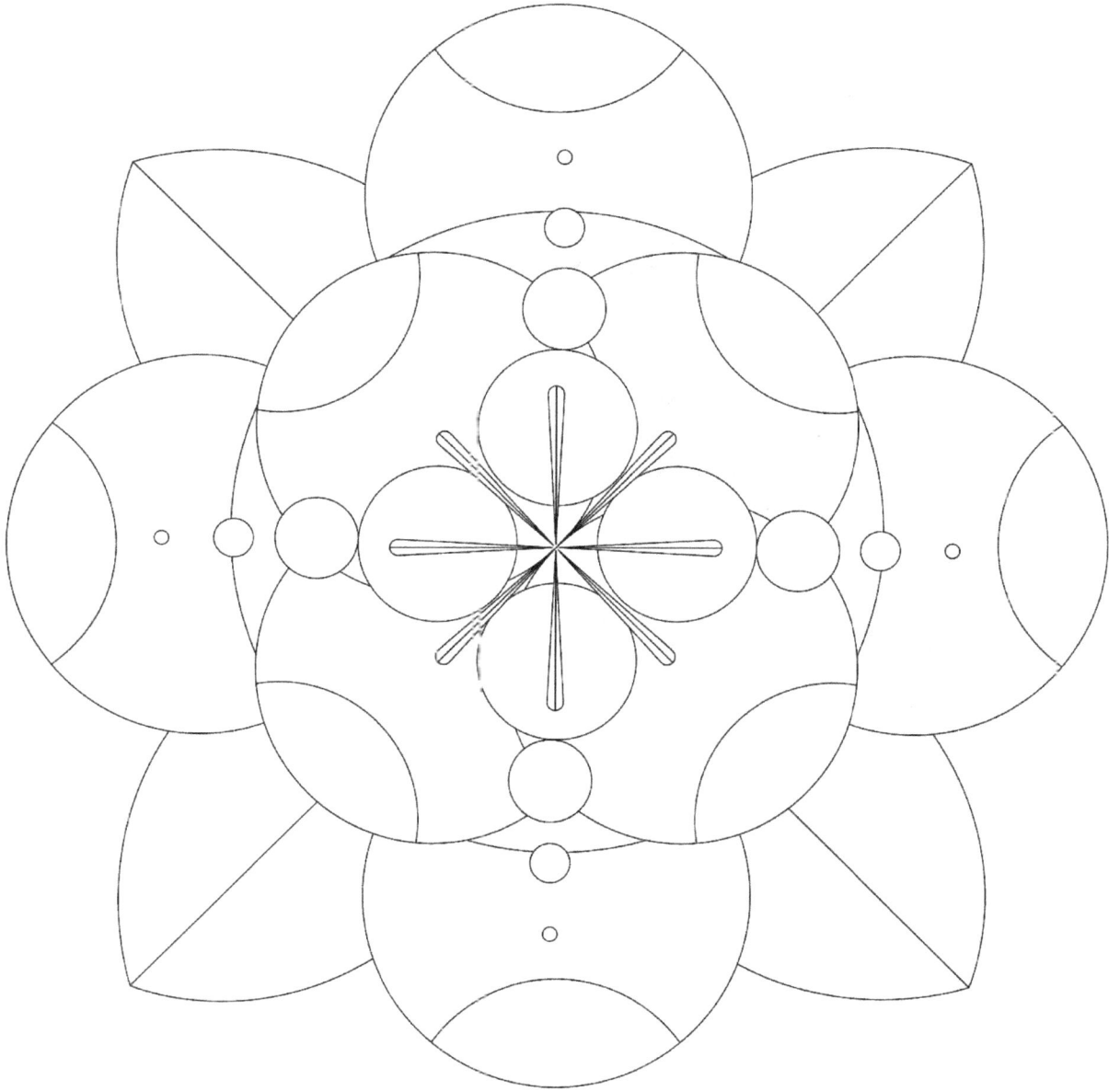

"Determine that the thing can and shall be done, and then we shall find the way."

President Abraham Lincoln

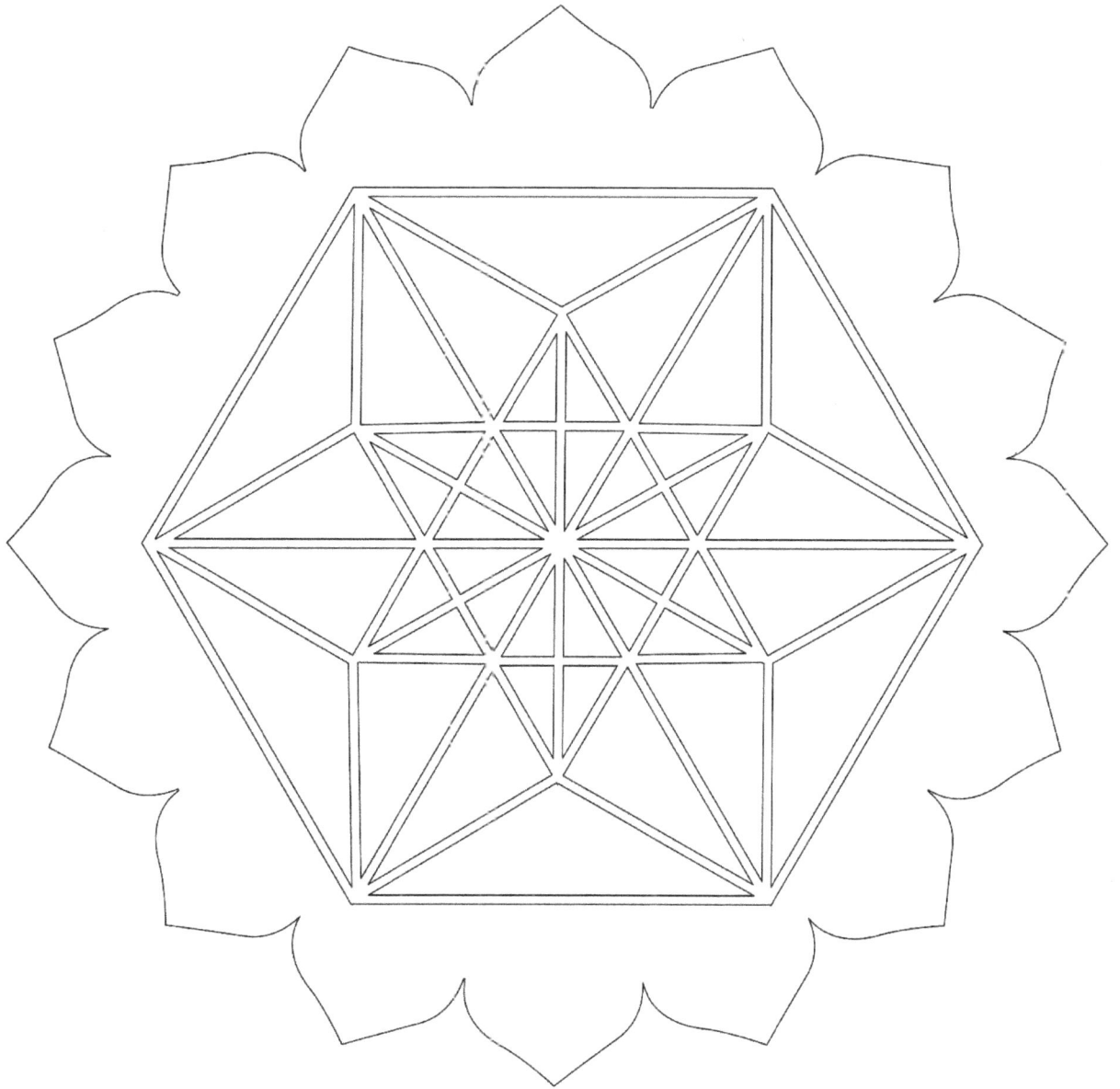

"You may have to fight a battle more than once to win it."

British Prime Minister Margaret Thatcher

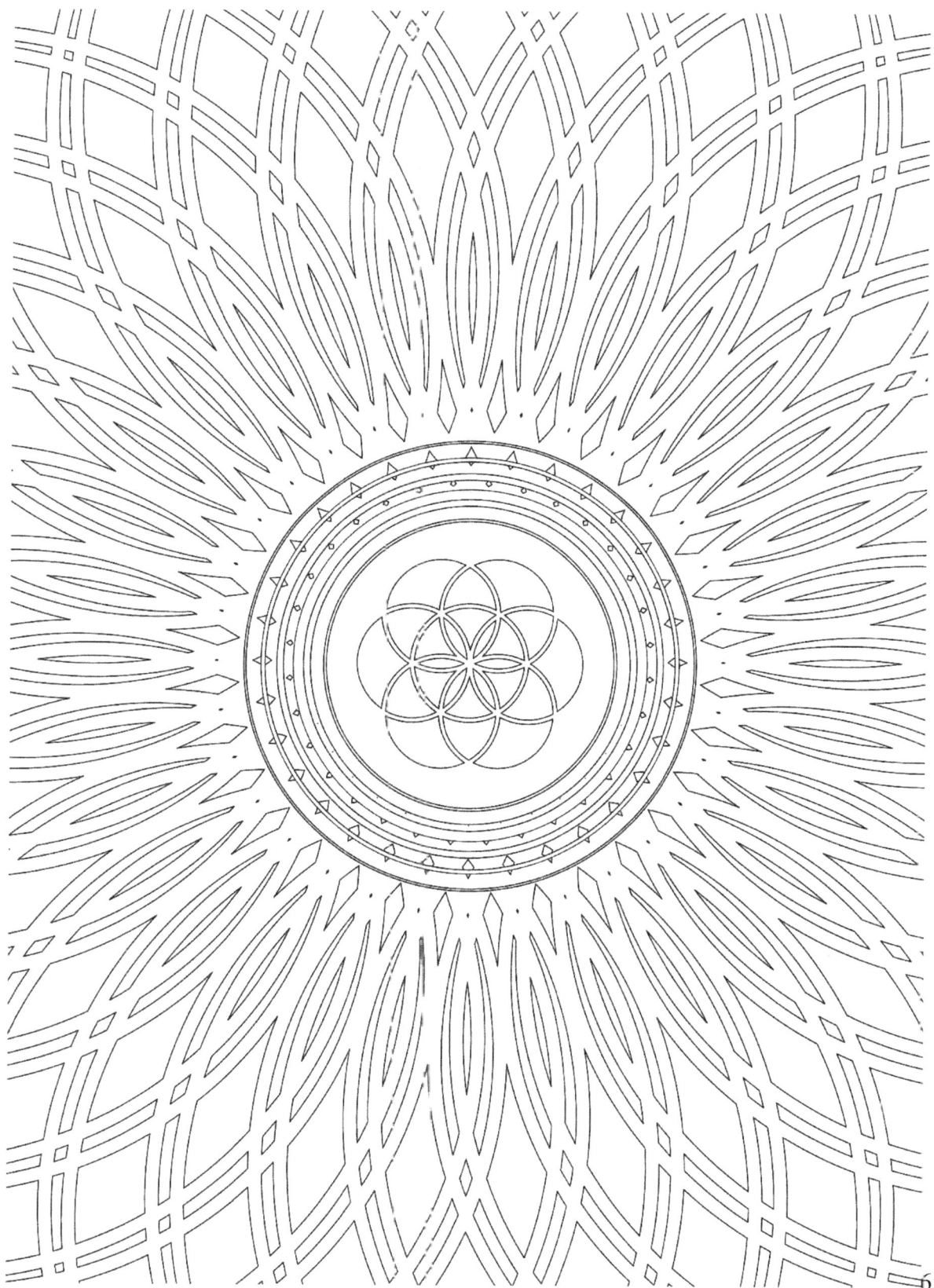

"Nothing worthwhile ever happens quickly and easily. You achieve only as you are determined to achieve; and as you keep at it until you have achieved."

Author Robert H. Lauer

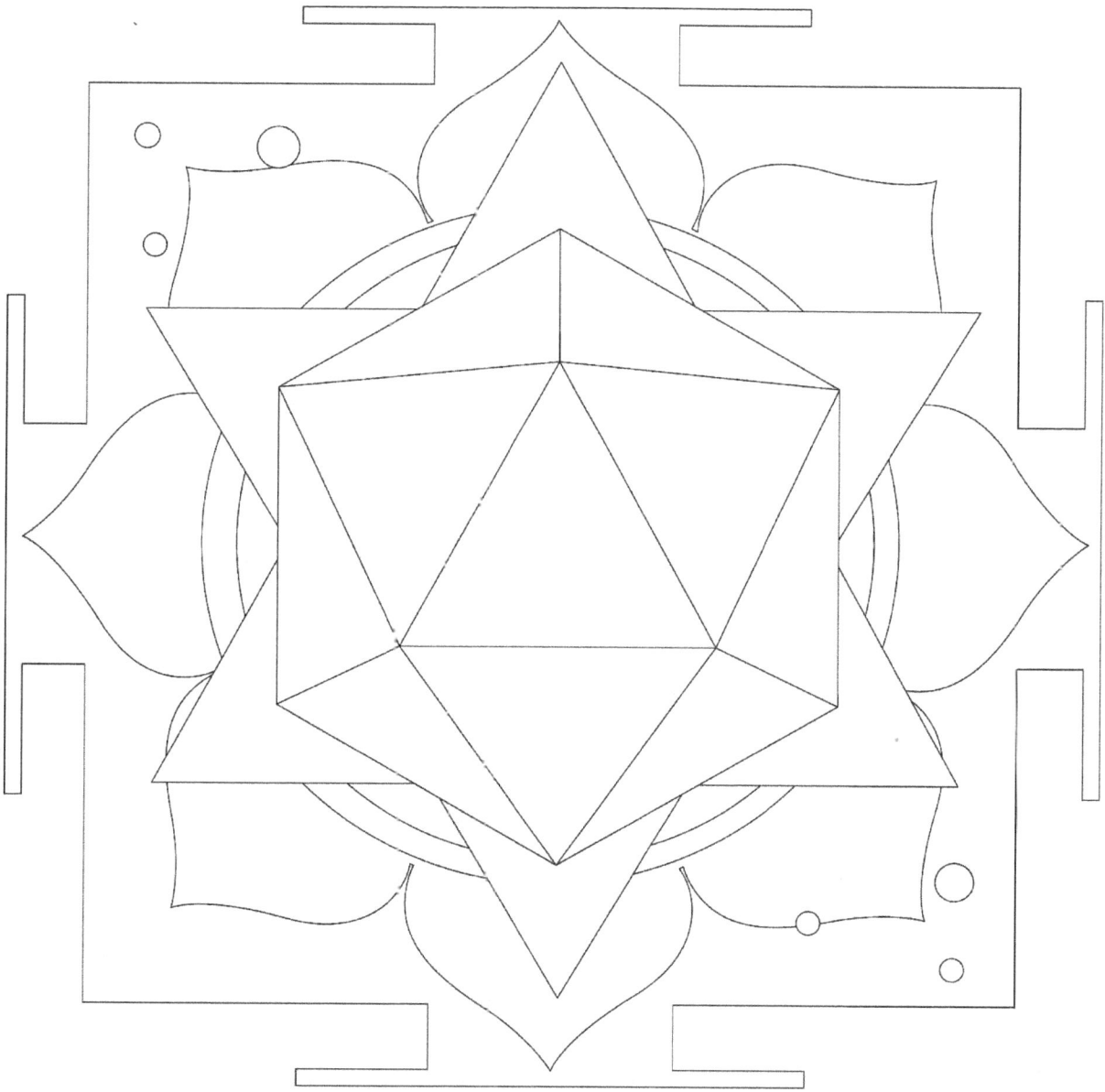

"The pessimist sees difficulty in every opportunity. The optimist sees opportunity in every difficulty."

Winston Churchill

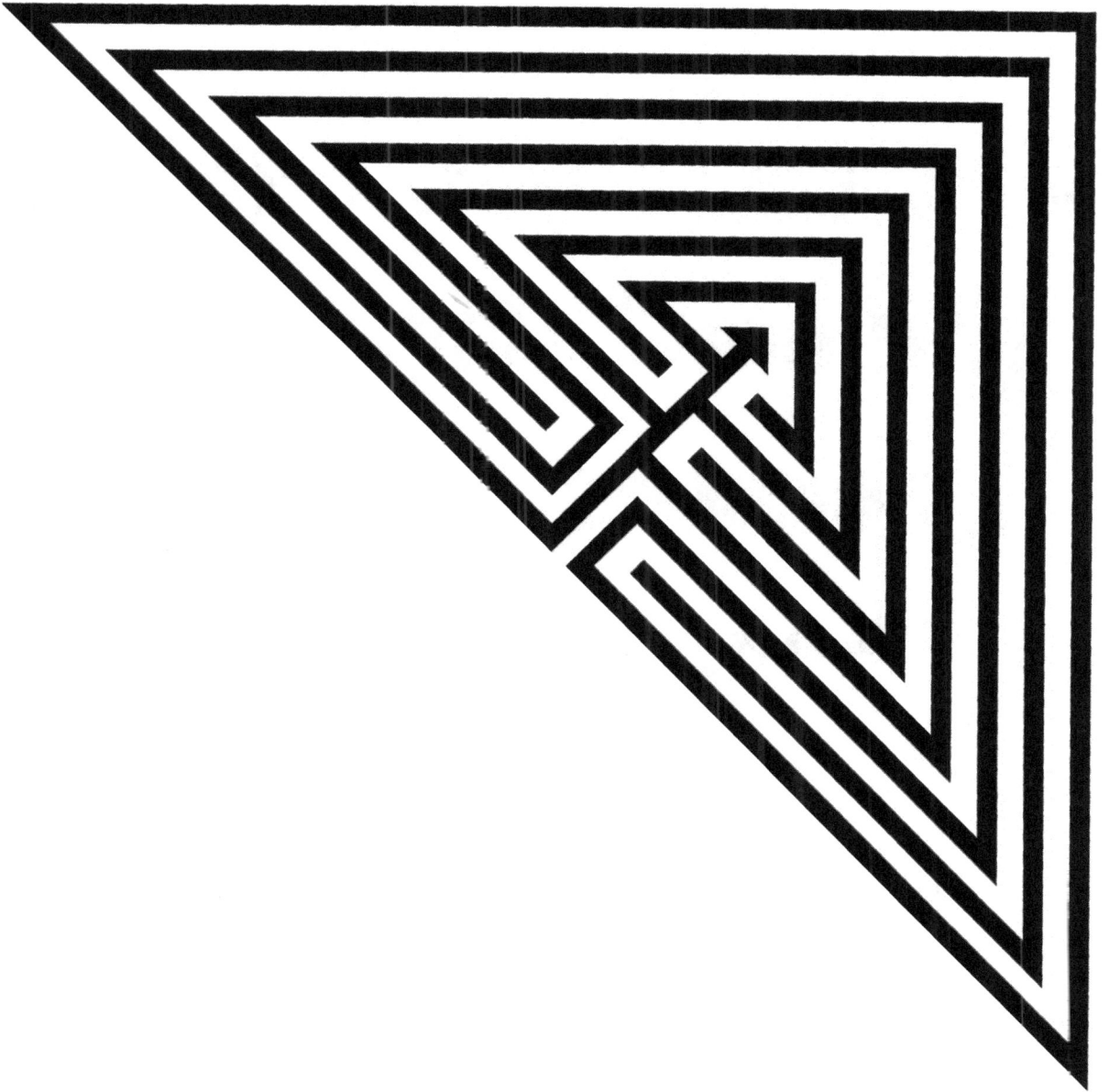

"Fake it until you make it!

Act as if you had all the confidence you require until it becomes your reality."

Brian Tracy

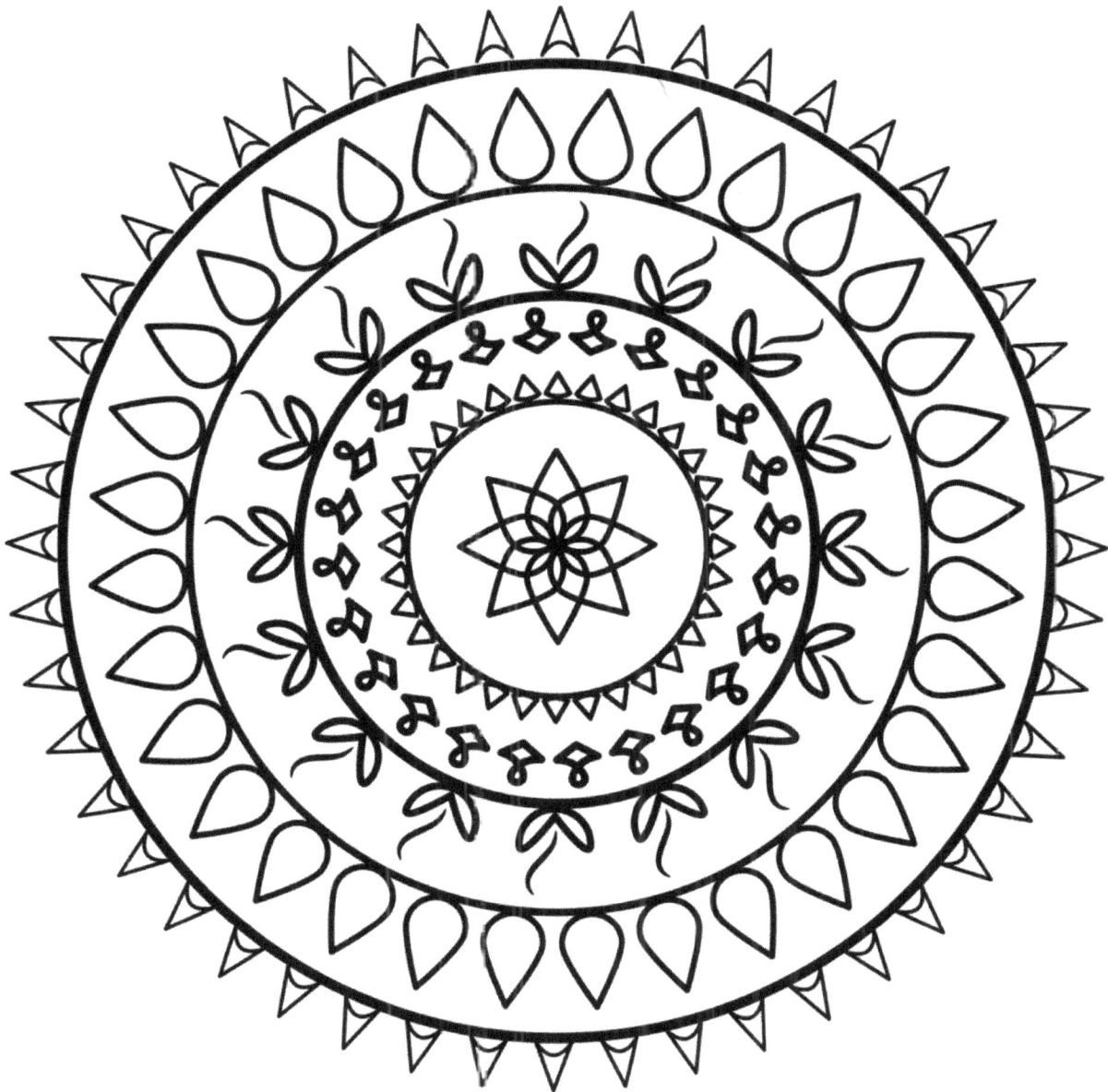

"One small crack does not mean that you are broken, it means that you were put to the test and you didn't fall apart."

Linda Poindexter

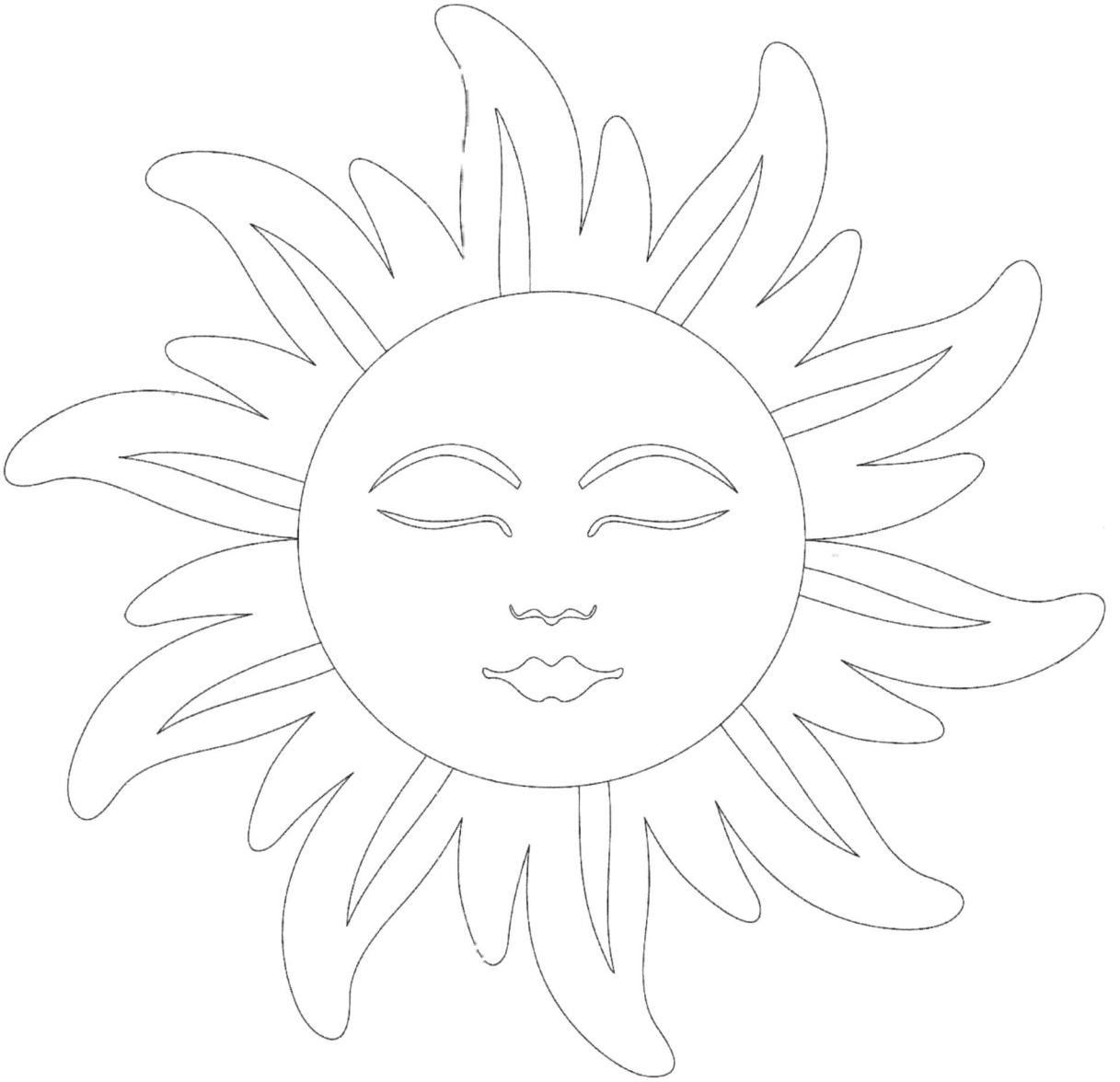

"We can't solve problems by using the same kind of thinking we used when we created them."

Albert Einstein

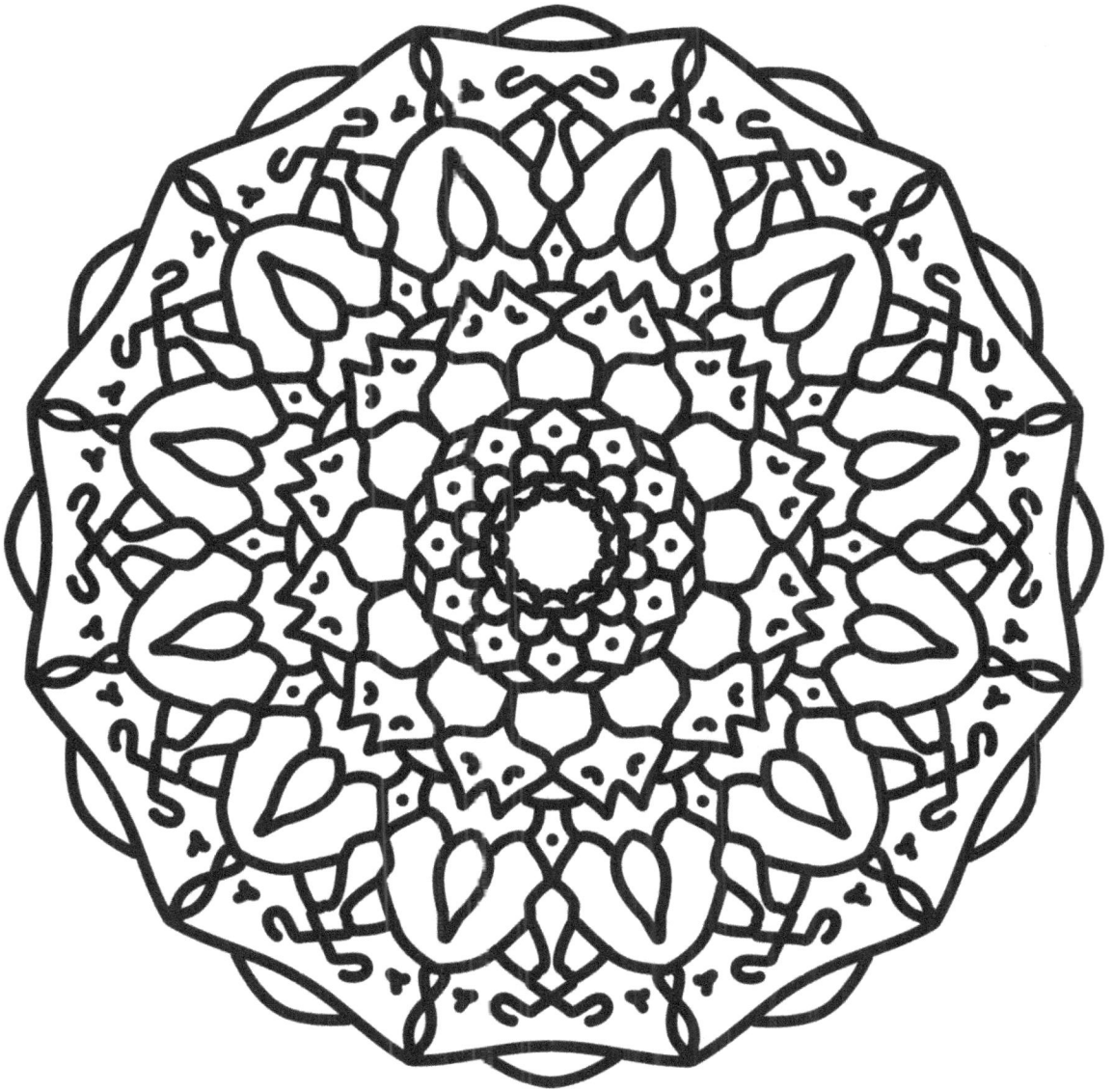

"Time is the coin of life. Only you can determine how it will be spent."

Carl Sandbur

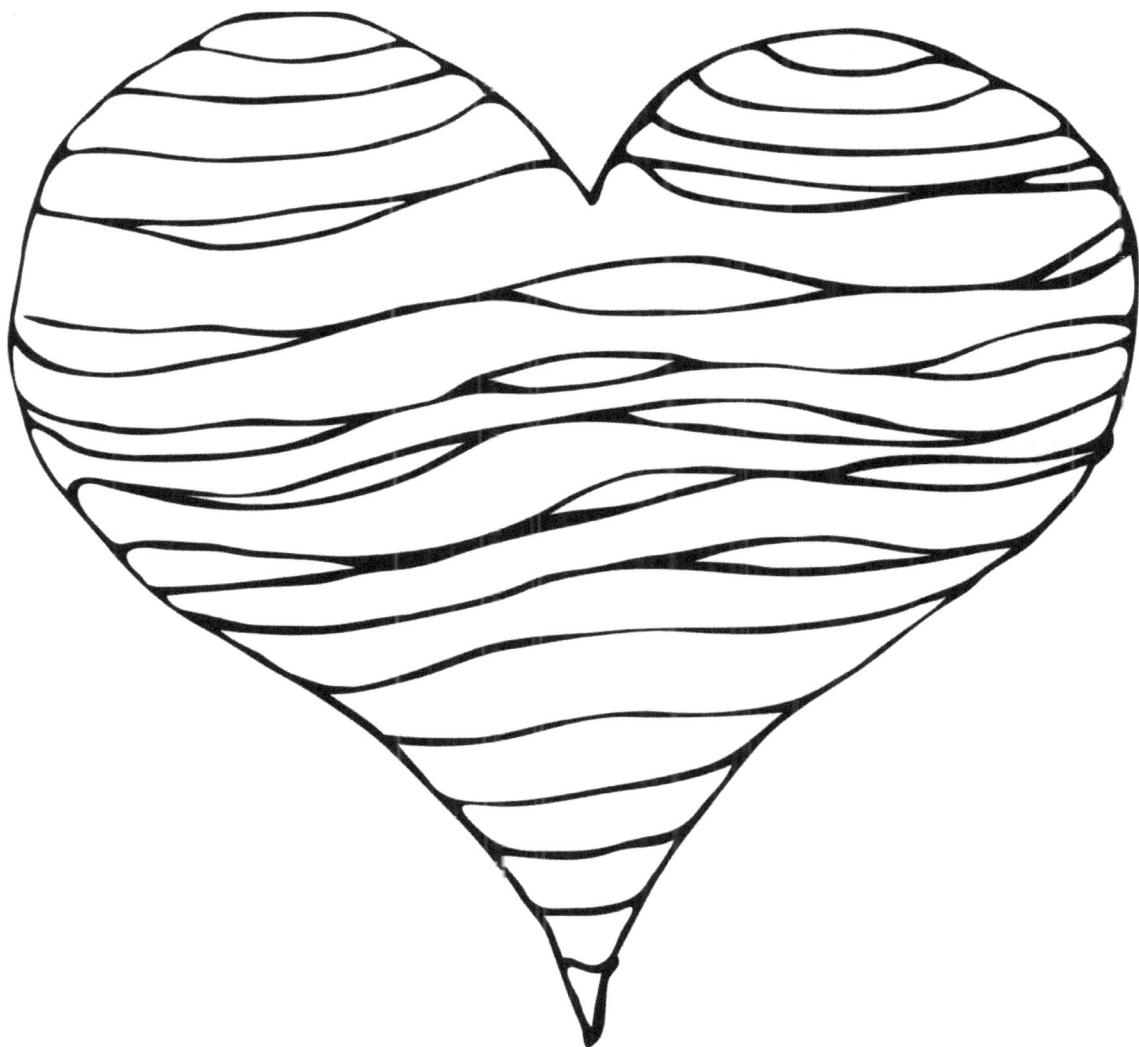

"We are what we repeatedly do. Excellence, therefore, is not an act but a habit."

Will Durant

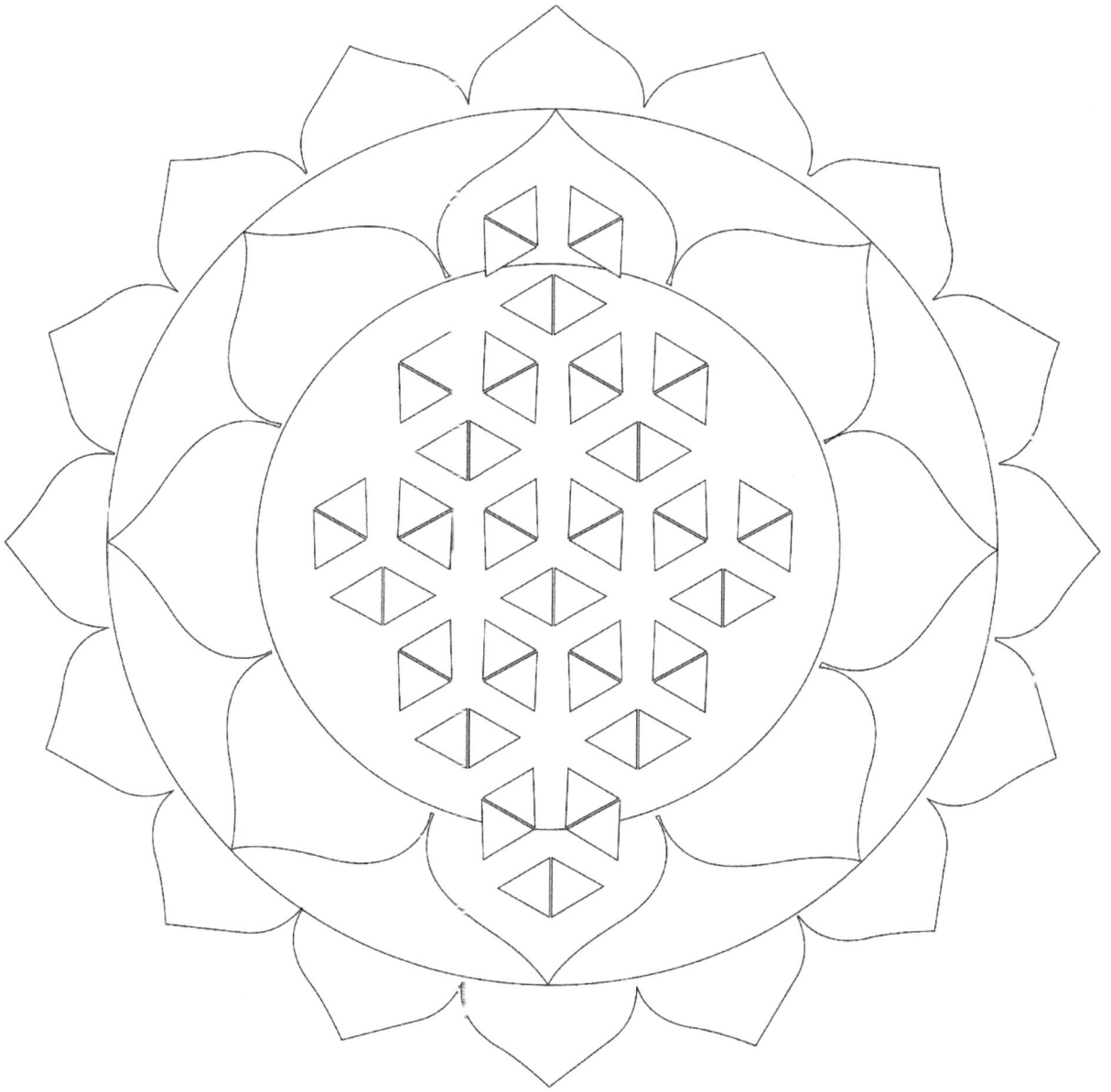

"Adopting the right attitude can convert a negative stress into a positive one."

Hans Selye

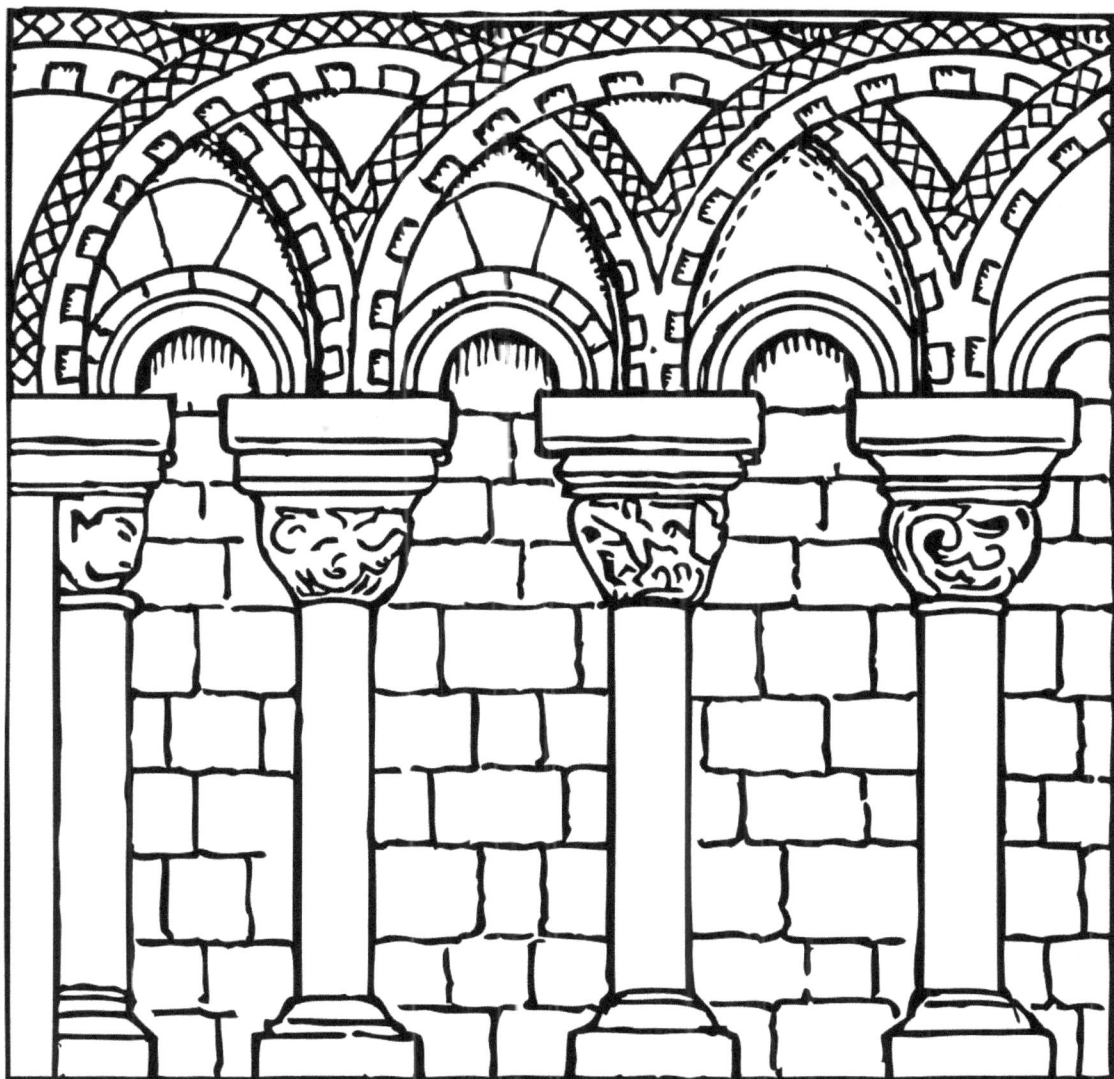

"There are far, far better things ahead than anything we leave behind."

C. S. Lewis

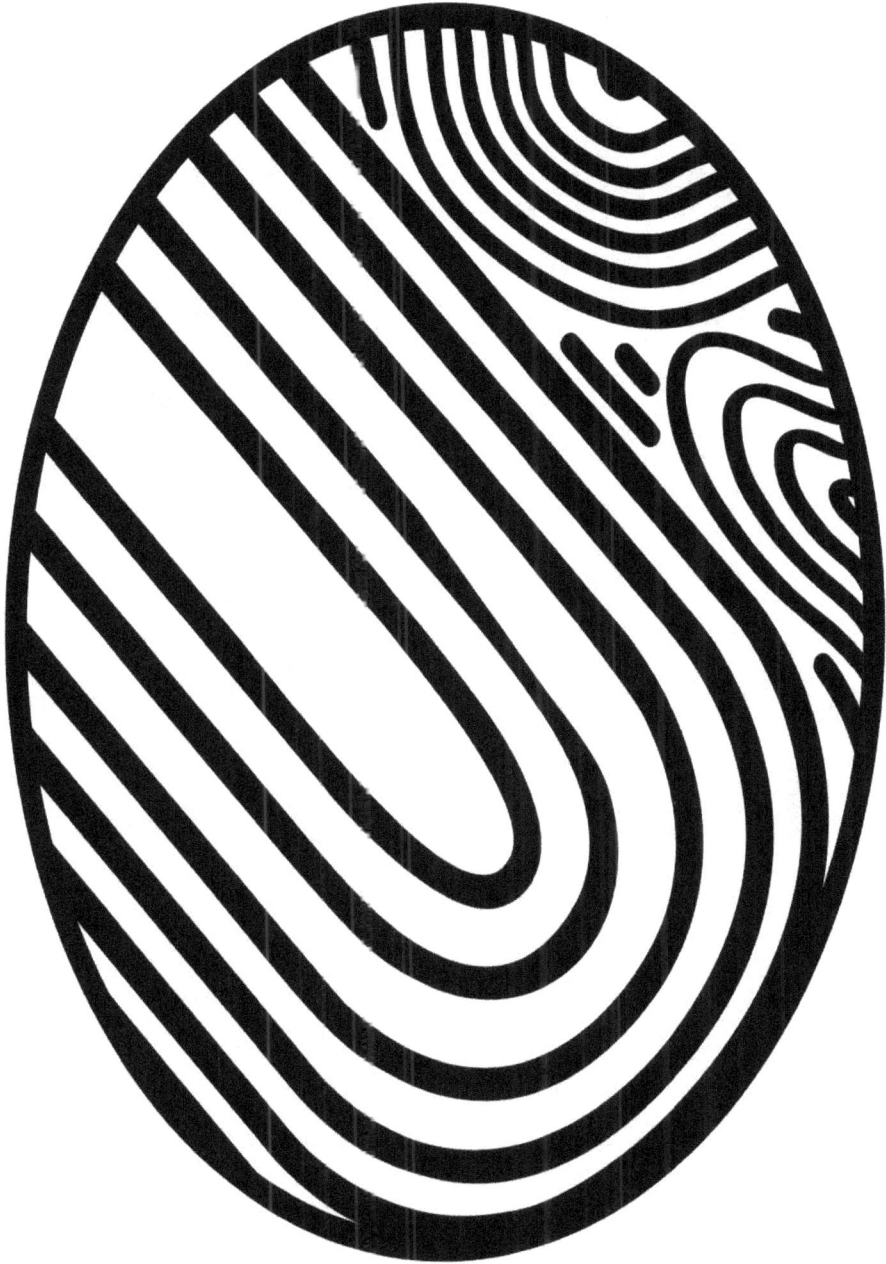

"Sometimes you can't see what is right in front of you but when you finally open your eyes you'll wonder why you didn't see it sooner."

Anonymous

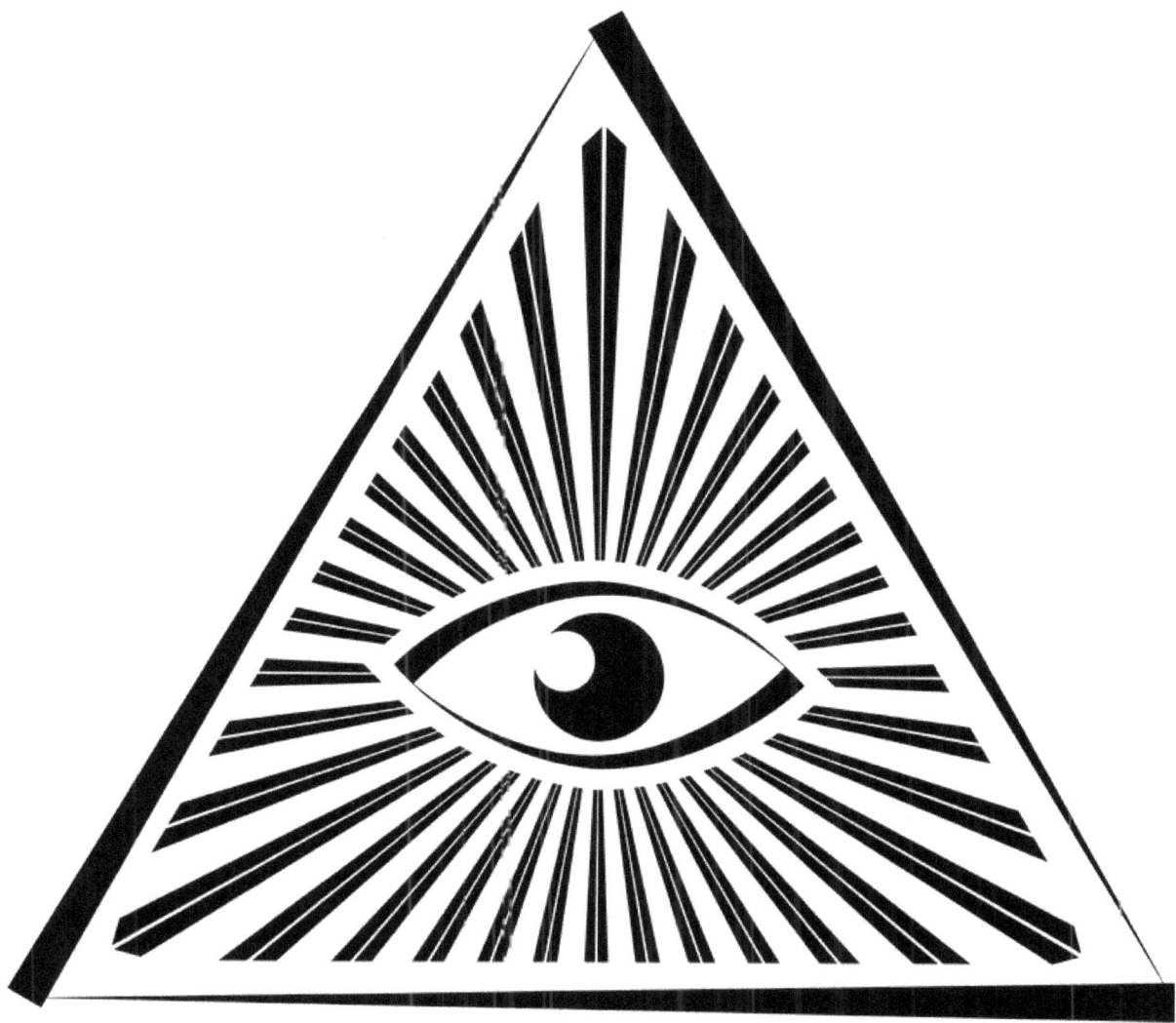

www.ingramcontent.com/pod-product-compliance
Lightning Source LLC
Chambersburg PA
CBHW081701270326
41933CB00017B/3234